The Human Side of Healing

A Master Manual on Professionalism, Patient Experience & Compassionate Care

From Treatment to Trust

For Doctors, Nurses & Healthcare Teams

Gerard Assey

The Human Side of Healing:

A Master Manual on Professionalism, Patient Experience & Compassionate Care

From Treatment to Trust For Doctors, Nurses & Healthcare Teams

By
Gerard Assey

Published by:
Gerard Assey
19/18, Palli Arasan Street
Anna Nagar East
Chennai - 600 102

ISBN: 978-81-69340-52-6

Table of Contents

DISCLAIMER

This book, ***"The Human Side of Healing: A Master Manual on Professionalism, Patient Experience & Compassionate Care—From Treatment to Trust,"*** is intended solely for educational, training, and informational purposes.

All names of individuals, healthcare professionals, patients, caregivers, hospitals, clinics, and organizations mentioned in this book are purely fictional. Any resemblance to actual persons, living or deceased, or to real institutions is entirely coincidental and unintentional.
The scenarios, case studies, and examples presented are created to reflect common situations in healthcare settings for the purpose of learning and professional development. They are not intended to depict or represent any specific individual, institution, or incident.

This book does not provide medical advice, diagnosis, or treatment recommendations. Healthcare professionals are advised to exercise their own clinical judgment and follow established medical guidelines, institutional protocols, and regulatory requirements while applying any concepts from this manual.
The author and publisher make no representations or warranties regarding the completeness, accuracy, or applicability of the content to specific situations. They shall not be held liable for any direct, indirect, incidental, or consequential outcomes arising from

the use or interpretation of the material contained in this book.

By using this book, readers acknowledge that the responsibility for applying the knowledge, tools, and techniques rests solely with them.
This work is a guide to enhance professionalism, communication, and patient experience, and is not a substitute for formal medical training, legal advice, or institutional policy.

PREFACE

There is a moment in every patient's journey that is rarely recorded in medical notes, never captured in diagnostic reports, and yet remembered for a lifetime.

It is the moment they ask themselves: *"Am I being cared for… or am I just being treated?"*

Modern medicine has achieved extraordinary milestones. Diseases once considered fatal are now manageable. Technology has brought speed, precision, and accuracy into diagnosis and treatment.

Yet, alongside these advancements, a quiet gap has widened—the gap between clinical excellence and human experience.

This book is born out of that gap.

"The Human Side of Healing: *A Master Manual on Professionalism, Patient Experience & Compassionate Care—From Treatment to Trust"* is not a critique of the medical profession. It is a call to elevate it. It recognizes the immense pressure, long hours, emotional burden, and life-and-death decisions that healthcare professionals carry every day. At the same time, it addresses a truth that cannot be ignored:

Patients may forget the exact treatment they received, but they will never forget how they were made to feel.

Healing, in its truest sense, is not complete without humanity.

WHY THIS BOOK MATTERS

Healthcare is not merely a system—it is an experience. Every interaction, whether at the reception desk, during a consultation, in a ward, or in a moment of crisis, shapes that experience.

- ✓ *A delayed appointment without communication creates anxiety.*
- ✓ *A rushed consultation creates doubt.*
- ✓ *A harsh tone creates fear.*
- ✓ *A lack of empathy creates distance.*

Conversely—

- ✓ *A kind word builds reassurance.*
- ✓ *A listening ear builds confidence.*
- ✓ *A respectful explanation builds trust.*

This manual is built on a simple but powerful belief: Professionalism in healthcare is not only about competence—it is about conduct, communication, and compassion.

WHO THIS BOOK IS FOR

This is a comprehensive, practical training manual designed for every individual who forms part of the healthcare ecosystem:

- ✓ *Doctors & Specialists – to strengthen patient communication, consultation quality, and trust-building*
- ✓ *Nurses & Paramedics – to enhance patient interaction, emotional support, and bedside care*
- ✓ *Reception & Front Desk Teams – to create strong first impressions and manage patient flow with professionalism*
- ✓ *Technicians & Support Staff – to understand their critical role in the patient experience*
- ✓ *Hospital Administrators & Leaders – to build systems and cultures centered on dignity and respect*

- ✓ *Medical Colleges & Training Institutions – as a structured curriculum for developing future-ready healthcare professionals*

HOW THIS BOOK SHOULD BE USED

This is not a book to be read once and set aside. It is designed to be used, practiced, and implemented.

Each chapter includes:

- ✓ *Real-life (fictional but realistic) scenarios drawn from everyday healthcare settings*
- ✓ *Reflection questions to challenge existing habits and assumptions*
- ✓ *Practical frameworks and communication models*
- ✓ *Role-play exercises for training sessions*
- ✓ *Ready-to-use tools and checklists for immediate application*

It can be used in multiple ways:

- ✓ *As a self-development guide for individual professionals*
- ✓ *As a training manual for hospitals and clinics*
- ✓ *As a workshop resource for group learning and role plays*
- ✓ *As a reference handbook for continuous improvement in patient care*

WHAT MAKES THIS MANUAL DIFFERENT

This is not a theoretical exploration of patient care. It is deeply practical, honest, and implementable.

It does not assume perfection. It acknowledges real-world challenges—overcrowded OPDs, time constraints, emotional fatigue, and systemic pressures. Yet, it demonstrates that even within these constraints, small, intentional changes can create extraordinary impact.

- ✓ *A pause before speaking.*
- ✓ *An explanation instead of instruction.*
- ✓ *A moment of eye contact.*
- ✓ *A tone that conveys respect.*

These are not additional tasks—they are transformational habits.

FROM TREATMENT TO TRUST

At its core, this book is about a shift:

From seeing patients as cases → to seeing them as people

From delivering treatment → to creating healing experiences

From managing processes → to building relationships

From authority → to trust

***Trust is the foundation of healthcare. Without it, even the best treatment is questioned. With it, even difficult journeys become bearable*.**

A FINAL WORD

Every healthcare professional enters this field with a purpose—to heal, to serve, to make a difference.

Over time, systems, pressures, and routines may dull that original intent. This manual is an invitation to rediscover it—not in grand gestures, but in everyday interactions.

Because in the end, the true measure of healthcare is not only in lives saved, but in lives touched.

May this book help transform every point of care into a point of connection. May it help move healthcare—from treatment… to trust.

Chapter 1:
The Silent Crisis in Healthcare

Bridging the Gap Between Clinical Excellence and Human Experience

---

There is a quiet contradiction at the heart of modern healthcare. On one hand, medicine has never been more advanced. Diagnostic tools are sharper, treatments more precise, survival rates higher. On the other hand, something deeply human seems to be slipping through the cracks—often unnoticed by those within the system, but profoundly felt by those who depend on it.

This is the silent crisis.

It does not show up in lab reports. It is not captured in discharge summaries. It rarely features in medical audits. Yet it is present in waiting rooms, in corridors, in the unspoken tension between caregivers and patients. It is the gap between what is medically delivered and what is emotionally experienced.

A patient may receive the correct diagnosis, the appropriate medication, and even a successful procedure—and still walk away dissatisfied, anxious, or even resentful. Not because the science failed, but because the *experience* did.

This chapter is not about blaming doctors, nurses, or healthcare systems. It is about recognizing a pattern that has quietly normalized itself—and beginning the work of changing it.

The Gap Between Clinical Expertise and Human Experience

Let us begin with an uncomfortable truth: clinical competence alone is no longer enough.

A highly skilled surgeon may perform a flawless operation, but if the patient feels ignored, confused, or disrespected throughout the journey, the overall perception of care is diminished. In today's world, patients do not separate "treatment" from "experience." To them, it is one continuous journey.

Consider the case of Mr. Ravi Menon, a 52-year-old corporate professional who visits a reputed hospital for chest discomfort. The cardiologist is brilliant—well-trained, experienced, and accurate in diagnosis. Within minutes, he identifies the issue as non-cardiac and reassures the patient medically. However, during the consultation, he barely looks up from his screen, interrupts Mr. Menon twice, and responds to questions with brief, technical answers.

From a clinical standpoint, the consultation is a success. From a human standpoint, it is not.

Mr. Menon leaves the hospital and tells his family, *"The doctor is knowledgeable, but I didn't feel comfortable. I don't think I'll go back."*

This is the gap.

It is not about lack of knowledge. It is about lack of *connection*.

And connection is not an "extra" in healthcare—it is central to healing.

Why Patients Remember Behavior More Than Treatment

Years later, when patients recount their medical experiences, they rarely begin with the diagnosis or the prescription. They begin with how they were treated as people.

"I was so scared, but the nurse held my hand."

"The doctor didn't even look at me."

"They made me feel like I was wasting their time."

"One kind word changed everything."

Human memory is wired to hold on to emotional experiences far more than technical details. In healthcare, where patients are often vulnerable, anxious, or in pain, this emotional imprint becomes even stronger.

Let us revisit the scenario introduced earlier:

Mr. Krishnan, a 64-year-old retiree, arrives at the outpatient department at 8:30 a.m. for a 9:00 a.m. appointment. Due to delays and overbooking, he is finally called in at 1:15 p.m. By this time, he is tired, hungry, and increasingly anxious about his health.

When he enters the consultation room, the doctor—already behind schedule—quickly reviews his reports, asks a few questions, and writes a prescription. The entire interaction lasts less than three minutes. There is no greeting, no acknowledgment of the long wait, no eye contact.

Medically, the diagnosis is correct. The treatment plan is appropriate.

But as Mr. Krishnan leaves, he mutters to his son, *"We waited all this time… and this is all we got?"*

Now pause and consider this carefully.

Ten years from now, Mr. Krishnan will not remember the exact medication prescribed that day. But he will remember how he felt—dismissed, unseen, unimportant.

This is not a minor issue. It directly affects:

- ✓ *Patient trust*
- ✓ *Treatment adherence*

- ✓ *Follow-up compliance*
- ✓ *Word-of-mouth reputation*

In many cases, it also determines whether a patient returns—or advises others to stay away.

The Rise of Mistrust Despite Medical Advancement

It is paradoxical. As healthcare has advanced scientifically, mistrust has grown socially.

Patients today are more informed, more aware, and more vocal than ever before. They have access to online reviews, medical information, and alternative opinions. But with this increased awareness has come increased scrutiny—and, often, skepticism.

Mistrust does not usually arise from a single major incident. It builds gradually through repeated small experiences:

- ✓ *Being spoken to abruptly*
- ✓ *Not being given clear explanations*
- ✓ *Feeling rushed during consultations*
- ✓ *Observing lack of coordination among staff*
- ✓ *Experiencing indifference at critical moments*

Let us consider another but very real-to-life situation.

Mrs. Latha Srinivasan brings her elderly father to the emergency department late at night. He is in visible discomfort. The staff is busy, and understandably so. However, no one explains what is happening. Forms are handed over without guidance. Questions are answered curtly. At one point, she is told, *"Please wait outside,"* without any indication of how long or why.

Her father receives appropriate medical care. He stabilizes.

But the experience leaves a mark.

A week later, when a neighbor asks for hospital recommendations, Mrs. Srinivasan hesitates. *"They are good doctors,"* she says, *"but I didn't feel they cared."*

This sentence captures the crisis perfectly.

Competence is acknowledged. Care is questioned.

And when care is questioned, trust begins to erode.

Understanding the Pressure on Healthcare Professionals

At this point, it is important to acknowledge the other side of the story.

Doctors, nurses, and paramedics operate under immense pressure. Long hours, high patient loads, administrative demands, emotional fatigue, and the constant weight of responsibility can gradually wear down even the most compassionate professionals.

What begins as dedication can slowly turn into detachment—not out of indifference, but as a coping mechanism.

A young doctor, Dr. Arjun, starts his career with enthusiasm and empathy. He spends time with patients, listens carefully, and explains conditions in detail. Over time, however, the realities of practice set in—overcrowded OPDs, time constraints, and institutional expectations.

Gradually, without even realizing it, his interactions become shorter, more transactional.

Not because he stopped caring—but because the system did not support him in sustaining that care.

This manual is not about ignoring these pressures. It is about equipping professionals to work effectively within them without losing the human touch.

Reframing the Problem: From Blame to Responsibility

The goal of this chapter is not to assign blame, but to create awareness.

The silent crisis exists not because healthcare professionals lack skill or intention, but because human experience has not been given equal importance as clinical outcomes.

The shift required is not massive, but it is meaningful.

It is the shift from:

- ✓ *Seeing patients as cases → to seeing them as people*
- ✓ *Delivering treatment → to creating an experience of care*
- ✓ *Managing time → to managing perception of time*
- ✓ *Communicating information → to connecting with individuals*

Action Framework: Closing the Gap in Daily Practice

Transformation begins with small, consistent actions. The following practices are simple, realistic, and immediately applicable—even in high-pressure environments.

1. The First 30 Seconds Matter Most

Every consultation should begin with presence. A brief pause, eye contact, and a simple acknowledgment can set the tone for the entire interaction.

Example:

"Good morning, Mr. Krishnan. I'm sorry you had to wait. Let's go through your concerns."

This takes less than 10 seconds—but changes everything.

2. Acknowledge the Patient's Experience

Patients do not expect perfection, but they do expect recognition.

Example:

"I understand you've been waiting for some time. Thank you for your patience."

This single sentence reduces frustration significantly.

3. Listen Without Interrupting (At Least Initially)

Allow the patient to speak for the first 30–60 seconds without interruption. This not only builds trust but often provides crucial information.

4. Replace Jargon with Clarity

Medical accuracy must be matched with understandable language.

Instead of: *"Your condition is non-cardiac in origin."*

Say: *"Your heart is fine. The discomfort is likely due to acidity or muscle strain."*

5. Close the Loop Before Ending the Consultation

Before the patient leaves, ensure clarity.

Example:

"Do you have any questions?"

"Would you like me to explain anything again?"

6. Small Gestures, Lasting Impact

A nod, a reassuring tone, a moment of patience—these are not time-consuming, but they are deeply impactful.

Training Reflection (For Individual & Group Sessions)

Take a moment to reflect on the opening scenario of Mr. Krishnan.

- ✓ What did the patient lose beyond time?

  He lost a sense of dignity, reassurance, and emotional comfort. He lost confidence in the system.

- ✓ What did the doctor lose without realizing?
  He lost the patient's trust, future loyalty, and possibly referrals. He also lost an opportunity to practice medicine in its fullest sense—not just as a science, but as a human service.

Closing Thought

Healthcare is one of the few professions where people come not by choice, but by need. They arrive with uncertainty, fear, and hope—often all at once.

In such moments, how they are treated matters as much as how they are treated medically.

The silent crisis will not be solved by technology, infrastructure, or policy alone. It will be addressed when healthcare professionals consciously bring back what has always been at the heart of healing:

Human connection!

The chapters that follow will not only explore this further but equip you with practical tools to make it a consistent part of everyday practice.

Chapter 2:
The Patient is Not a Case File

Humanizing the Journey from Entry to Exit

There is a moment, often brief but deeply defining, when a patient steps into a healthcare facility. It may be at the reception desk, outside an emergency room, or in the quiet uncertainty of an outpatient corridor. In that moment, the individual is not thinking in clinical terms. There is no awareness of protocols, workflows, or hospital pressures. What exists instead is a mixture of concern, fear, urgency, and hope.

Yet, somewhere between registration numbers, case sheets, and diagnostic codes, this human reality is often reduced to a file.

A name becomes a token number. A person becomes a "case." A story becomes a set of symptoms.

This chapter addresses a foundational shift that must occur if healthcare is to regain its human core: the patient must never be reduced to a case file.

The Invisible Shift: From Person to Process

In busy healthcare environments, standardization is necessary. Systems, formats, and documentation are essential for efficiency and safety. However, what begins as a system for order can quietly become a system of detachment.

- ✓ A nurse calls out, *"Next case."*
- ✓ A doctor asks, *"What's the issue?"* without looking up.
- ✓ A technician says, *"Sit there,"* pointing without explanation.

None of these are acts of intentional disrespect. They are habits—formed over time, reinforced by pressure, and rarely questioned.

But for the patient, these moments accumulate into a powerful impression: *"I am not being seen as a person."*

Let us consider a simple but revealing scenario.

Scenario: The Fever That Became Fear

Meera, a young mother, rushes into a clinic with her five-year-old son, Aarav, who has been running a high fever since the previous night. She is anxious, sleep-deprived, and visibly worried.

At the nursing station, she explains, *"My son has had a fever since last night, and he's not eating…"*

Without looking up fully, the nurse responds, *"Wait outside."*

No tone of reassurance. No explanation of what will happen next. No acknowledgment of her concern.

Meera sits down, clutching her child, her mind racing. *Is it something serious? Why didn't the nurse ask more questions? How long will we have to wait? Should I have gone somewhere else?*

Every passing minute amplifies her anxiety—not because of the fever alone, but because of the *silence* around it.

Now consider an alternative approach.

The same nurse, under the same workload, responds differently:

"Alright, I understand you're worried. Let me just check a few details. The doctor will see you shortly—there may be a short wait of about 15–20 minutes. If the fever increases or if he becomes uncomfortable, please let me know immediately."

The medical process remains unchanged. But the experience is transformed.

This is the difference between processing a case and caring for a person.

Understanding the Emotional State of Patients and Caregivers

To humanize care, one must first understand the emotional landscape of those seeking it.

Patients do not arrive in a neutral state. Even in routine visits, there is an undercurrent of concern. In more serious situations, that concern becomes fear, and sometimes even panic.

Caregivers, in particular, carry a dual burden. They are not only worried about the patient but are also responsible for making decisions, understanding information, and managing logistics. This creates a heightened emotional state that can easily tip into frustration if not handled with sensitivity.

Consider Mr. Dinesh, accompanying his elderly mother for a cardiac evaluation. He has taken time off work, arranged transportation, and is already under pressure. When he is met with unclear instructions and delayed responses, his frustration builds quickly—not because he is unreasonable, but because he is overwhelmed.

In such situations, even a neutral response from staff can be perceived as dismissive.

This is a critical insight for healthcare professionals: Patients and caregivers do not interpret interactions objectively—they interpret them emotionally.

The Psychology of Vulnerability

At the core of every patient interaction lies one powerful factor: vulnerability.

When individuals enter a healthcare setting, they are stepping into an environment where they have limited control and limited understanding. They are dependent on professionals not just for treatment, but for clarity, reassurance, and guidance.

This vulnerability manifests in different ways:

- ✓ *Some patients become quiet and withdrawn*
- ✓ *Others ask repeated questions*
- ✓ *Some may appear demanding or impatient*
- ✓ *Caregivers may become anxious or even confrontational*

These behaviors are often misunderstood.

A patient who asks the same question multiple times is not being difficult—they are seeking reassurance.

A caregiver who appears impatient is not necessarily disrespectful—they are afraid.

Let us look at another situation.

Scenario: The "Difficult" Patient

Mrs. Farzana Begum, a 58-year-old woman, is admitted for a minor surgical procedure. She repeatedly asks the nurse, *"When will the doctor come? Is everything okay? Will it be painful?"*

The nurse, already attending to multiple patients, responds curtly, *"Please wait. The doctor will come."*

Mrs. Begum continues to ask similar questions over the next hour, growing increasingly anxious.

From the nurse's perspective, this is a "difficult patient."

From the patient's perspective, this is a moment of uncertainty and fear.

Now imagine a different response.

The nurse sits beside her for a brief moment and says, *"I understand you're feeling anxious. The doctor is expected in about 30 minutes. The*

procedure is routine, and we'll be with you throughout. If you feel worried, you can call me anytime."
That one minute of engagement can reduce repeated interruptions, ease anxiety, and create a sense of safety.
Understanding vulnerability is not about spending more time—it is about using time more effectively.

Reframing the Patient Journey
To truly humanize healthcare, one must begin to see the patient journey not as a series of clinical steps, but as a series of emotional transitions.
From the moment a patient enters the facility to the moment they leave, they move through stages:

- ✓ *Arrival with uncertainty*
- ✓ *Waiting with rising anxiety*
- ✓ *Consultation with expectation*
- ✓ *Diagnosis with emotional impact*
- ✓ *Exit with either clarity or confusion*

At each stage, the role of the healthcare professional is not just to perform a task, but to guide the patient through that emotional transition.
This requires awareness, intention, and a consistent approach.

Action Plan: Bringing Humanity Back into Everyday Practice
Humanizing care does not require additional infrastructure or extended consultation times. It requires a shift in awareness and a few deliberate practices.
Every interaction must begin with acknowledgment. A simple recognition of the patient's presence and concern creates an immediate connection. Even in

high-pressure environments, this can be achieved with a brief but genuine response.

Explanation must become a standard practice, not an exception. Patients should never be left guessing what will happen next. Even a short sentence explaining the process can significantly reduce anxiety.

Tone must be consciously managed. In healthcare, words carry weight, but tone carries meaning. A neutral sentence delivered without warmth can be perceived as cold or dismissive.

Staff must learn to identify emotional cues. A patient who looks anxious, a caregiver who seems restless, a child who appears frightened—these are not peripheral observations. They are central to effective care.

Finally, closure must be intentional. Before a patient leaves any interaction point, they should have clarity on what comes next. Uncertainty is one of the biggest contributors to dissatisfaction.

The Empathy Mapping Tool: Seeing Beyond the Symptoms

To make this approach practical and trainable, healthcare teams need a simple way to understand patients beyond their medical condition. One of the most effective tools for this is Empathy Mapping.

This is not a theoretical exercise. It is a practical framework that can be used in training sessions, team discussions, and even individual reflection.

Let us take the earlier example of Meera and her child.

An empathy map for Meera would look like this when explored in a training setting:

What is she *thinking*?

She is worried about her child's health. She is questioning whether she acted quickly enough. She is unsure about what will happen next.
What is she *feeling*?
Anxiety, fear, helplessness, and urgency.
What is she *saying*?
"My child has had a fever… he's not eating… I'm really worried."
What is she *doing*?
Holding her child closely, looking around for reassurance, repeatedly checking for attention.
What does she *need*?
Reassurance, clarity, timely attention, and a sense that someone is in control.
When healthcare professionals begin to see patients through this lens, their responses naturally change.
Instead of saying, *"Wait outside,"* the response becomes, *"I understand you're concerned. Let me guide you through what happens next."*
Empathy mapping can be practiced during training sessions using real or fictional scenarios. Over time, it becomes instinctive.

A Culture Shift, Not a One-Time Effort
Humanizing healthcare is not about isolated acts of kindness. It is about creating a culture where every member of the team—from reception to senior consultants—understands their role in shaping the patient experience.
It requires leadership commitment, consistent training, and ongoing reinforcement.
But most importantly, it requires a shift in mindset.
Patients are not interruptions to workflow. They are the reason the system exists.

They are not case files to be processed. They are individuals seeking help at a moment when they are most vulnerable.

Closing Reflection

Think back to a time when you or someone close to you needed medical care.

What stood out? Was it the accuracy of the diagnosis—or the way someone spoke, listened, or reassured?

The answer to that question is at the heart of this chapter.

When healthcare professionals begin to see beyond the file and connect with the person, something powerful happens.

Trust is built. Anxiety is reduced. Outcomes improve—not just medically, but emotionally. And in that moment, healthcare returns to what it was always meant to be:

Not just a science of treatment, but a practice of care.

Chapter 3: The Cost of Poor Professional Behavior

What Healthcare Loses When Conduct Falls Short

In healthcare, outcomes are measured in numbers—recovery rates, infection rates, readmission rates. These are necessary and non-negotiable. Yet there is another set of outcomes, less visible but equally decisive, that determine whether a hospital is trusted, recommended, and respected.

These outcomes are shaped not by clinical skill alone, but by professional behavior.

A dismissive tone, a careless remark, an avoidable delay without explanation—each of these may appear minor in isolation. But together, they create a pattern. And patterns, over time, become reputation, culture, and risk.

This chapter examines the real cost of poor professional behavior—not as a moral argument, but as an operational reality that affects patients, institutions, and healthcare professionals themselves.

When Trust Begins to Erode

Trust is the foundation on which all medical care rests. Without it, even the most accurate diagnosis can be questioned, and the most effective treatment can be resisted.

Trust is not built in a single interaction. It is built in small, consistent moments—how a patient is greeted, how questions are answered, how uncertainty is handled. Conversely, it is also lost in small, repeated lapses.

Consider the experience of Mr. Joseph D'Souza, a 47-year-old school teacher who visits a well-known hospital for persistent headaches. During his first consultation, the doctor appears hurried and does not fully address his concerns. When Mr. D'Souza tries to ask additional questions, he is told, *"Let's not overthink this. Just follow the prescription."*

He leaves with medication, but also with doubt.

A week later, when the symptoms persist, he hesitates to return. Instead, he consults another doctor at a smaller clinic, where the interaction is slower, more conversational, and more reassuring. The second doctor confirms the same diagnosis and prescribes a similar treatment plan.

Yet Mr. D'Souza chooses to continue with the second doctor. The difference is not medical. It is relational.

The first doctor did not lose the patient because of incompetence, but because of a perceived lack of engagement. And once trust is weakened, it is difficult to rebuild.

For healthcare institutions, this translates into more than a single lost patient. It affects retention, referrals, and long-term credibility.

From Dissatisfaction to Disputes: The Legal Dimension

It is often assumed that legal cases in healthcare arise primarily from clinical errors. While clinical negligence is certainly a factor, a significant number of disputes originate from something less obvious: communication breakdown and perceived indifference.

When patients or families feel unheard, disrespected, or kept in the dark, their response can escalate from dissatisfaction to confrontation.

Let us consider the case of Mrs. Kavita Rao, whose husband is admitted for a routine surgical procedure. The surgery is successful, but during recovery, he develops a minor complication that requires extended observation.

The medical team manages the complication appropriately. However, no one clearly explains the situation to the family. Updates are brief, technical, and inconsistent. At one point, a junior staff member casually mentions, *"There was a small issue during recovery, but it's under control."*

The word "issue" triggers alarm.

Mrs. Rao begins to question what is being hidden. She seeks clarification but receives fragmented responses from different staff members. Anxiety turns into suspicion.

By the time a senior doctor sits down to explain the situation in detail, the damage is already done. The family has lost confidence. They begin to document interactions, seek external opinions, and consider legal action.

What could have been a routine recovery with a minor complication becomes a case of distrust.

The lesson here is critical:

When communication is weak, even good clinical care can appear questionable.

Clear, timely, and empathetic communication is not just a courtesy—it is a protective factor against legal risk.

Reputation in the Digital Era: Every Experience is Public

There was a time when patient experiences were shared within small circles—family, friends, neighbors. Today, every experience has the potential to become public.

A single review on a digital platform can reach hundreds, sometimes thousands, of prospective patients. And unlike clinical outcomes, which are difficult for the public to assess, behavior is immediately visible and easily judged.

Consider Sunita Verma, a young professional who visits a diagnostic center for a routine test. The process is delayed, the staff appears indifferent, and her questions are answered impatiently.

Later that evening, she writes a detailed review online:

"The test was fine, but the staff was rude and unhelpful. No one explained anything. I felt completely ignored."

Within days, the review receives multiple views and responses. Some users share similar experiences. The perception begins to form—not necessarily about the quality of medical care, but about the quality of interaction.

For a healthcare institution, this is a critical distinction.

Patients may not have the expertise to evaluate clinical decisions, but they are fully equipped to evaluate how they are treated.

Reputation today is shaped as much by patient experience narratives as by medical outcomes. And once a negative perception takes hold, it requires significant effort to correct.

The Internal Cost: Staff Burnout and Cultural Decline

While the external consequences of poor professional behavior are significant, the internal impact is equally serious—and often overlooked.

Workplace culture in healthcare is deeply interconnected. The way professionals treat patients is often a reflection of how they experience their own work environment.

In settings where communication is rushed, appreciation is rare, and pressure is constant, a gradual erosion of empathy can occur. What begins as fatigue can evolve into detachment.

Let us look at Nurse Priya, who has been working in a busy hospital ward for several years. She is competent, dedicated, and initially known for her warmth with patients. Over time, however, the demands increase—long shifts, high patient loads, and limited support.

She begins to feel that no matter how much she does, it is never enough.

Gradually, her interactions change. She becomes more task-focused, less conversational. When patients ask repeated questions, she feels irritated rather than empathetic. This is not a failure of character. It is a sign of burnout.

Now consider the impact.

Patients begin to perceive her as indifferent. Complaints increase. Supervisors address the complaints, but without addressing the underlying workload or emotional strain.

The cycle continues.

This is how poor professional behavior and burnout reinforce each other. A strained environment leads to reduced empathy, which leads to negative patient experiences, which in turn increase pressure and dissatisfaction within the team.

Breaking this cycle requires recognizing that professional behavior is not just an individual responsibility—it is a cultural outcome.

A Practical Shift: From Reaction to Responsibility

If the costs are so high, why does poor professional behavior persist?

In most cases, it is not due to a lack of awareness, but a lack of structured focus. Clinical training is rigorous and detailed. Behavioral training, however, is often informal, inconsistent, or absent.

To address this, healthcare institutions must move from expecting professionalism to training and reinforcing it systematically.

At an individual level, professionals can begin with a simple but powerful shift: moving from reaction to responsibility.

Instead of reacting to patient behavior—whether anxious, impatient, or repetitive—there must be a conscious effort to respond with clarity and composure.

For example, when a caregiver repeatedly asks for updates, the instinctive reaction may be irritation. The responsible response, however, is to recognize the underlying anxiety and address it proactively.

A doctor might say, *"I understand you're concerned. Let me explain where we are and what to expect in the next few hours."*

This does not require additional time. It requires intentional communication.

Action in Practice: Small Changes, Measurable Impact

In training environments, it is important to translate these insights into daily practice.

A hospital that implemented a simple protocol—ensuring that every patient receives a brief explanation during delays—observed a noticeable reduction in complaints. The protocol did not change scheduling or workload. It changed communication.

In another setting, junior doctors were trained to summarize the consultation at the end in plain language. This reduced follow-up confusion and improved patient satisfaction scores.

These are not large-scale reforms. They are focused behavioral adjustments that produce measurable outcomes.

Rebuilding Culture from Within

Sustainable change cannot rely on individual effort alone. It must be supported by leadership and embedded in the culture of the institution.

Senior doctors, administrators, and department heads play a critical role in setting expectations—not just for clinical excellence, but for professional conduct.

When respectful communication, patient acknowledgment, and team collaboration are consistently modeled at the top, they become normalized throughout the organization.

Conversely, when dismissive behavior is tolerated or overlooked, it spreads.

Culture is not defined by policies. It is defined by what is practiced daily.

Closing Reflection

Every interaction in healthcare carries weight. Not all of them are remembered, but many of them shape perception, trust, and decision-making.

When professional behavior falls short, the cost is not immediate or always visible. It appears over time—in lost trust, in strained relationships, in reputational damage, and in the quiet exhaustion of those within the system.

But the reverse is equally true.

When professionalism is practiced consistently—through respectful communication, clear explanations, and genuine engagement—the impact is profound.

Patients feel safe. Families feel reassured. Teams function more effectively. And healthcare, in its truest sense, begins to fulfill not just its clinical purpose, but its human promise.

The chapters ahead will build on this foundation, moving from awareness to structured skill-building—so that professionalism is not left to chance, but becomes a deliberate and reliable part of everyday care.

Chapter 4: What True Professionalism Looks Like

Beyond Degrees: The Daily Practice of Behavior, Tone and Presence

---

There is a moment of quiet realization that comes to many patients after a consultation. It is not about the diagnosis, nor the prescription. It is something more subtle. They say, "That doctor is good," or sometimes, "I didn't feel comfortable there."

What informs that judgment is rarely a technical evaluation. It is an evaluation of professionalism—not as defined in textbooks, but as experienced in real time.

In healthcare, qualifications open the door. Professionalism determines whether people walk through it again.

A degree certifies knowledge. Professionalism reveals character in action.

This chapter examines what professionalism truly looks like—not as an abstract ideal, but as a set of observable, trainable behaviors that shape patient experience every single day.

Beyond Degrees: The Unspoken Evaluation

Patients cannot assess your clinical reasoning. They do not see the years of study, the complexity of diagnosis, or the precision of your decision-making. What they do see is how you carry yourself.

They notice whether you look at them or at your screen.

They notice whether you listen or interrupt.
They notice whether your tone is calm or hurried.
They notice whether they feel safe asking a question—or hesitant.

This is the unspoken evaluation happening in every interaction.

Let us consider Dr. Mehul Shah, a highly qualified specialist with an impeccable academic record. His consultations are efficient, accurate, and fast. However, he rarely pauses to acknowledge the patient. His tone is neutral, sometimes abrupt. Questions are answered, but not invited.

Across the corridor, Dr. Anita Varghese, equally competent, practices differently. She begins each consultation with a brief acknowledgment, listens without interruption for the first minute, and explains her diagnosis in simple language before writing the prescription.

Both doctors treat correctly.

But patients consistently say, *"I prefer Dr. Anita."*

This preference is not accidental. It is built on behavior, tone, and presence.

Professionalism, therefore, is not an additional skill layered on top of medicine. It is the manner in which medicine is practiced.

Understanding Presence: The Most Overlooked Skill

Presence is often misunderstood as simply being physically available. In reality, it is about being mentally and emotionally attentive in the moment.

A doctor may be in the room, but mentally occupied with the next patient. A nurse may be performing a task, but emotionally disengaged due to fatigue. Patients sense this immediately.

Consider Mr. Iqbal Khan, who visits a clinic for a follow-up. As he explains his symptoms, the doctor continues typing, occasionally nodding but not making eye contact. When Mr. Khan finishes, the doctor responds with a diagnosis that may well be correct.

Yet Mr. Khan hesitates and says, *"Doctor, I'm not sure if you understood what I was trying to say."*

What happened here is not a failure of knowledge. It is a failure of presence.

Now imagine the same interaction with a small shift. The doctor pauses typing for a moment, looks at Mr. Khan, and says, *"Go ahead, I'm listening."* Even if the typing resumes later, that initial moment of attention establishes connection.

Presence does not require more time. It requires intentional focus.

The Five Pillars of Medical Professionalism

To make professionalism practical and consistent, it must be broken down into core elements that can be understood, practiced, and evaluated. These form the five pillars that support every meaningful patient interaction.

Respect: The Foundation of Every Interaction

Respect in healthcare is not limited to polite language. It is demonstrated through how patients are acknowledged, how their time is valued, and how their dignity is preserved.

A patient who has waited for hours deserves acknowledgment. A caregiver who asks repeated questions deserves patience. A junior staff member deserves to be spoken to with the same courtesy as a senior colleague.

Consider Mrs. Nalini Krishnamurthy, an elderly patient who struggles to hear clearly. During her consultation, she repeatedly asks the doctor to repeat instructions. The doctor, pressed for time, responds with visible impatience.

Mrs. Nalini leaves the room embarrassed and confused.

Now consider an alternative approach. The doctor leans slightly forward, speaks a little louder but gently, and says, *"No problem, I'll explain it again. Take your time."*

The clinical outcome remains unchanged. But the experience is transformed.

Respect is not about grand gestures. It is about small, consistent signals that say, *"You matter."*

In practice, this means consciously slowing down tone even when time is limited, addressing patients by name, and avoiding dismissive language—even unintentionally.

Communication: The Bridge Between Knowledge and Understanding

Medical knowledge is only useful when it is understood.

Communication is where many healthcare interactions succeed or fail. It is not enough to provide information. The information must be clear, relevant, and tailored to the patient's level of understanding.

Let us look at Ramesh, a daily wage worker diagnosed with hypertension. The doctor explains the condition using technical terms and prescribes medication. Ramesh nods, collects the prescription, and leaves.

Two weeks later, he returns with uncontrolled blood pressure. When asked, he admits he stopped taking the medication because he felt better.

The issue here is not non-compliance. It is miscommunication.

Now imagine the doctor had said, *"This is a long-term condition. Even if you feel fine, you must continue the medicine daily. If you stop, the problem can return silently."*

That one sentence could have changed the outcome.

Effective communication is not about speaking more. It is about ensuring understanding. It involves checking whether the patient has grasped the key message, inviting questions, and avoiding assumptions.

Responsibility: Owning the Patient Journey

Responsibility in healthcare extends beyond performing a specific task. It includes ensuring that the patient is guided through the entire process without confusion or neglect.

A common breakdown occurs when responsibility is fragmented.

A patient is sent from one department to another without clear instructions. A test is advised, but no one explains where to go. A discharge is given, but follow-up steps are unclear.

Each individual may have performed their role correctly. Yet the patient experiences the system as disorganized.

Consider Mr. Suresh Patel, who is advised to undergo a series of tests. He moves from the consultation room to the billing counter, then to the diagnostic area, receiving minimal guidance at each step. By the end of the process, he is frustrated and exhausted.

Now imagine a coordinated approach where one staff member says, *"I'll guide you through the next steps. First, please go to billing, and then they will direct you to diagnostics. If you have any difficulty, come back to me."*

Responsibility here is not about doing everything. It is about ensuring continuity of care.

Professionals who take ownership of the patient journey reduce confusion, improve efficiency, and build trust.

Empathy: Understanding Without Assumption

Empathy is often misunderstood as sympathy or emotional involvement. In a professional setting, empathy is the ability to understand the patient's emotional state and respond appropriately—without becoming overwhelmed by it.

It is the difference between saying, *"You'll be fine,"* and saying, *"I understand this is worrying. Let me explain what we're seeing."*

Consider Arun, a young man awaiting biopsy results. He appears calm but asks very few questions. The doctor assumes he is not concerned and provides a brief explanation.

In reality, Arun is deeply anxious but unsure how to express it.

An empathetic approach would involve observing this silence and gently inviting conversation: *"I notice you're quiet. Is there anything specific you're worried about?"*

This opens the door for honest communication.

Empathy is not about dramatic expressions. It is about attunement—noticing what is said, and what is not.

Reliability: Consistency That Builds Confidence

Reliability is the pillar that sustains trust over time. It is reflected in consistency—keeping commitments, maintaining standards, and being dependable.

A doctor who is frequently late without explanation, a nurse who provides inconsistent information, or a system that changes processes unpredictably—all of these erode reliability.

Consider Dr. Fernandes, who is known for his clinical expertise but is often delayed by several hours. Patients continue to come because of his reputation, but frustration builds with each visit.

Eventually, even loyal patients begin to look for alternatives—not because they doubt his skill, but because they cannot depend on his schedule.

Reliability does not mean perfection. It means predictability and accountability.

If delays are unavoidable, they must be communicated. If processes change, they must be explained. When patients know what to expect, they feel more in control.

Bringing the Pillars into Daily Practice

Professionalism becomes meaningful only when it is practiced consistently.

In a busy outpatient department, a doctor may not have the luxury of extended consultations. Yet professionalism can still be demonstrated through brief but intentional actions.

A nurse managing multiple patients can still maintain a calm tone. A receptionist handling a long queue can still acknowledge waiting patients with a simple update.

The goal is not to create ideal conditions, but to practice professionalism within real constraints.

A Practical Integration Exercise

During training sessions, healthcare teams can be asked to reflect on a recent interaction that did not go well. Instead of assigning blame, the situation can be analyzed through the five pillars.

1. *Was respect maintained?*
2. *Was communication clear?*
3. *Was responsibility taken for guiding the patient?*
4. *Was empathy demonstrated?*
5. *Was reliability upheld?*

This structured reflection turns everyday experiences into learning opportunities.

Closing Perspective

Professionalism in healthcare is often spoken about, but rarely defined in practical terms. It is not a single act, nor a personality trait. It is a series of choices made repeatedly, often under pressure.

It is the decision to pause and acknowledge.

- ✓ *To explain instead of assume.*
- ✓ *To listen instead of rush.*
- ✓ *To guide instead of redirect.*
- ✓ *To remain steady, even when the environment is not.*

When these choices become consistent, professionalism is no longer an expectation. It becomes a habit.

And when professionalism becomes a habit, something remarkable happens.

Patients begin to feel not just treated—but truly cared for.
That is the standard this manual seeks to build.

Chapter 5: Medical Etiquette – The Forgotten Skill

Small Behaviors, Lasting Impressions

In the practice of medicine, there are skills that are formally taught, rigorously examined, and continuously updated. Then there are skills that are assumed, rarely trained, and quietly neglected—yet they shape the patient's experience more immediately than any clinical decision.

Medical etiquette belongs to the second category.

It is not written in prescriptions, nor documented in case sheets. It is expressed in how a patient is received, how a question is heard, how a concern is answered, and how a conversation is closed. It is the difference between a consultation that feels transactional and one that feels reassuring.

Over time, as systems become busier and consultations more compressed, etiquette is often the first casualty. Not because it is unimportant, but because it is misunderstood as optional.

It is not optional.

In reality, etiquette is the visible face of professionalism. It is what patients encounter before, during, and after every clinical interaction. When done well, it creates ease, trust, and clarity. When ignored, it creates distance, doubt, and dissatisfaction.

The First Moment: Greeting as a Clinical Tool

A greeting may seem like a social formality, but in healthcare, it carries clinical significance. It sets the tone for the interaction and signals whether the patient is entering a space of attention or indifference.

Consider Mr. Balasubramanian, who enters a consultation room after waiting for over an hour. The doctor, focused on the screen, says without looking up, *"Yes, what's the problem?"*

The consultation has begun—but the connection has not.

Now imagine a different beginning.

The doctor looks up briefly, makes eye contact, and says, *"Good morning, Mr. Balasubramanian. Please come in. I'm sorry for the wait—how can I help you today?"*

The difference in time is negligible. The difference in experience is significant.

A proper greeting does three things at once. It acknowledges the patient's presence, it establishes respect, and it invites communication. Without it, the interaction begins with a subtle imbalance—the patient feels like an interruption rather than a priority.

In high-volume settings, even a brief acknowledgment—using the patient's name if available—can create a sense of being seen. This is not about extending consultation time. It is about using the first few seconds with intention.

Body Language: What You Say Without Speaking

Patients observe far more than what is spoken. They read posture, eye contact, gestures, and movement—often unconsciously, but with strong emotional impact.

A doctor leaning slightly forward signals engagement. A nurse standing with crossed arms may unintentionally signal distance. A clinician who continues to look at a screen while a patient speaks conveys divided attention, even if the intention is efficiency.

Let us revisit a common situation.

Scenario: The Divided Consultation

Dr. Nikhil Rao is consulting in a busy outpatient department. As Mrs. Leela Iyer begins to describe her symptoms, he starts typing into the computer. He occasionally nods, asks short questions, and continues entering data.

Mrs. Iyer hesitates midway. She slows down, unsure if she should continue speaking. When she finishes, she says softly, *"Doctor, I'm not sure if I explained it properly."*

From Dr. Rao's perspective, he has captured all necessary information. From Mrs. Iyer's perspective, she is not confident she was heard.

Now consider a small but meaningful adjustment.

As Mrs. Iyer begins speaking, Dr. Rao pauses typing for the first 30–40 seconds, looks at her, and listens fully. Once she completes her initial explanation, he says, *"Alright, I understand. Let me just note this down,"* and resumes typing.

This sequence changes the perception entirely.

The lesson here is not to stop documentation, but to sequence attention—first listen, then record. Body language, when aligned with intention, reinforces trust. When misaligned, it creates doubt.

Tone of Voice: The Emotional Carrier of Words

Words convey information. Tone conveys meaning.

A sentence spoken in a calm, respectful tone can reassure. The same sentence, delivered hurriedly or sharply, can create discomfort—even if the words are technically correct.

Consider the difference between:

"You need to take this medicine regularly."

and

"You need to take this medicine regularly, alright? It will help control the condition."

The second carries reassurance. The first may sound directive.

Tone becomes especially important in moments of stress—when patients are anxious, when caregivers are asking repeated questions, or when delays are unavoidable.

Let us consider Mr. Arvind, who approaches the nurse's station to ask about his wife's test results. The nurse, already managing multiple tasks, responds, *"We will inform you when it's ready."*

The information is correct. The tone, however, feels dismissive.

Now imagine the same response delivered differently:

"It should be ready shortly. I understand you're waiting—please give us a little more time, and we'll update you."

The content is identical. The experience is not.

Tone requires conscious regulation, especially under pressure. It is not about being overly soft or artificial. It is about being clear, calm, and respectful—even when busy.

Listening Without Interruption: The Discipline of Attention

Listening is often assumed, but rarely practiced fully.

In many consultations, patients are interrupted within the first few seconds. The intention is usually efficiency—to guide the conversation quickly toward diagnosis. However, premature interruption often leads to incomplete understanding and repeated clarifications later.

Consider Shalini, who visits a clinic for recurring abdominal discomfort. As she begins to explain, the doctor interrupts after a few words and asks, *"Is it after food?"*

She nods, but the fuller context of her symptoms is lost. The consultation proceeds, but key details are missed, leading to a less effective treatment plan.

Now imagine a different approach.

The doctor allows Shalini to speak uninterrupted for the first minute. She explains not only the timing of the discomfort but also associated symptoms and lifestyle factors. The doctor then asks targeted questions.

The overall consultation time may remain the same, but the quality of information is significantly better.

Listening without interruption is not about extending time. It is about allowing the patient to complete their narrative before directing it.

Patients who feel heard are more cooperative, more trusting, and more likely to follow advice.

A Practical Shift: From Habit to Intentional Practice

Medical etiquette often fails not because professionals are unaware, but because habits take over under pressure.

To change this, etiquette must be brought into conscious practice until it becomes natural again.

A simple internal framework can help guide every interaction:

- ✓ *Before speaking, acknowledge.*
- ✓ *While listening, focus.*
- ✓ *While responding, explain.*
- ✓ *Before closing, confirm.*

These are not additional tasks. They are refinements of existing ones.

Role Play Exercise: The "Wrong Way vs Right Way" Consultation

To make etiquette practical and trainable, it must be experienced, not just discussed. One of the most effective methods is structured role play.

Let us take a common outpatient scenario.

The "Wrong Way" Consultation

A patient enters. The doctor continues typing and says, *"Yes, tell me."*

The patient begins speaking. The doctor interrupts within seconds, asks rapid questions, and continues looking at the screen.

When the patient hesitates, the doctor fills the silence with assumptions.

The prescription is written quickly. The doctor says, *"Take this and come back if needed."*

The patient leaves with limited clarity and low confidence.

The "Right Way" Consultation

The patient enters. The doctor looks up briefly and says, *"Good morning. Please have a seat."*

The doctor pauses typing and allows the patient to explain the concern without interruption.

After the initial explanation, the doctor says, *"Alright, I understand. Let me ask a few questions,"* and proceeds with focused inquiry.

While documenting, the doctor occasionally maintains eye contact and acknowledges responses.

Before concluding, the doctor explains the diagnosis in simple terms, outlines the treatment, and asks, *"Do you have any questions?"*

The patient leaves with clarity and reassurance.

Training Application

During workshops, participants can enact both versions of the consultation. Observers can be asked to reflect not on medical accuracy, but on how the interaction felt.

This creates immediate awareness of the impact of small behavioral differences.

Repeated practice helps professionals internalize these behaviors until they become part of their natural style.

Closing Perspective

Medical etiquette is often described as "basic," but its impact is profound.

It does not require advanced training, additional time, or complex systems. It requires awareness, intention, and consistency.

- ✓ *A greeting that acknowledges.*
- ✓ *A posture that listens.*
- ✓ *A tone that reassures.*
- ✓ *A pause that allows expression.*

These are not extras in healthcare. They are essentials.

When practiced consistently, they transform the consultation from a clinical exchange into a human connection.
And in that connection, healing begins—not just through treatment, but through trust.

Chapter 6: Time Management vs Patient Respect

Balancing Efficiency with Dignity in Every Minute

Time is one of the most strained resources in healthcare. Clinics run behind schedule, emergencies disrupt carefully planned appointments, and doctors are often required to move between responsibilities with little margin for delay. In such an environment, time management becomes a necessity.

Yet, for the patient, time is experienced very differently.

A delay is not just a delay. It is uncertainty. It is anxiety. It is the feeling of being overlooked.

This chapter addresses a tension that exists in almost every healthcare setting: the conflict between operational time pressures and the patient's need for respect. The goal is not to eliminate delays—that would be unrealistic—but to manage them in a way that preserves trust and dignity.

Why Delays Happen: A Realistic View from Inside the System

To address delays effectively, one must first understand their causes. Most delays in healthcare are not the result of negligence. They are the result of complexity.

A doctor may be delayed because a previous patient required more time than expected. A consultation that was meant to last ten minutes extends to twenty

because of unexpected complications. A routine case suddenly becomes serious. An emergency case arrives without warning and must be prioritized.
There are also systemic factors. Overbooking is often done with the intention of maximizing access. Administrative processes take longer than anticipated. Coordination between departments may not always be seamless.
Consider Dr. Vivek Menon, who begins his outpatient consultations at 9:00 a.m. By 9:30 a.m., he is already behind schedule. The first patient required extended counseling after receiving difficult news. The second patient had multiple co-morbidities that needed careful evaluation. By mid-morning, the delay has accumulated.
From Dr. Menon's perspective, every delay has a reason. From the patient's perspective in the waiting area, there is only one reality: *"The doctor is late."*
This difference in perception is where frustration begins.

The Patient's Experience of Waiting
Waiting in a healthcare setting is not passive. It is emotionally active.
A patient sitting in a waiting area is not simply passing time. They are thinking, worrying, observing, and often imagining worst-case scenarios. Every passing minute without information amplifies uncertainty.
Let us consider Mrs. Geetha Raman, who arrives for a consultation regarding persistent fatigue. She has taken leave from work, arranged transportation, and mentally prepared for the visit. Her appointment is at 10:00 a.m.

By 10:30, there is no update. By 11:00, she begins to feel restless. By 11:30, she is frustrated. Not because of the delay alone, but because she does not know *why* she is waiting or *how long* it will continue.

At 11:45, she approaches the reception desk and is told, *“Doctor is late. Sit.”*

The response is brief, factual, and dismissive.

Now compare this with a different approach.

At 10:15, the receptionist announces, *“There has been a delay due to an emergency case. The doctor is expected to be available in about 30–40 minutes. We appreciate your patience.”*

At 10:45, an update is provided again.

The delay remains the same. But the experience is entirely different.

Patients are far more accepting of delays when they are informed, acknowledged, and respected.

Communication: The Difference Between Frustration and Patience

The way delays are communicated often determines how they are perceived.

A delay without explanation feels like neglect. A delay with explanation feels like a circumstance.

Let us revisit the scenario:

“Doctor late. Sit.”

This statement conveys information, but it lacks context and courtesy. It leaves the patient with unanswered questions and a sense of dismissal.

Now consider:

“Doctor is delayed by 20 minutes due to an emergency. Thank you for your patience.”

This statement does more than inform. It explains, acknowledges, and appreciates.

The difference lies in three elements: clarity, reason, and respect.

Let us take another example.

Mr. Prakash, waiting for a follow-up consultation, approaches the desk after a long wait. The staff member, overwhelmed by the crowd, responds sharply, *"We will call you when it's your turn."*

Mr. Prakash returns to his seat, irritated.

Now imagine the same situation handled differently.

"I understand you've been waiting. There are two patients ahead of you. It should take about 20 minutes. Thank you for your patience."

The second response takes only a few seconds longer, but it restores a sense of order and respect.

Communication during delays is not an additional responsibility. It is an essential part of patient care.

Structuring OPD Flow: Bringing Order to the Experience

While communication addresses perception, structure addresses the root of the issue.

Outpatient departments often struggle not because of the volume of patients alone, but because of how that volume is managed.

A well-structured flow does not eliminate delays entirely, but it reduces unpredictability and improves overall efficiency.

Let us consider a common situation.

In a busy clinic, patients are scheduled at ten-minute intervals. However, actual consultations vary widely. Some take five minutes, others take twenty. Over time, the schedule becomes misaligned with reality.

Patients continue to arrive based on their appointment times, but the system is already running behind.

Now imagine a different approach.

Appointments are categorized based on expected consultation time. Follow-up visits are scheduled differently from first-time consultations. Buffer slots are built into the schedule to accommodate unexpected delays.

Additionally, a staff member is assigned to monitor patient flow and provide real-time updates.

In such a system, delays may still occur, but they are managed proactively rather than reactively.

A Practical Example of Flow Improvement

At a mid-sized clinic, repeated complaints about waiting time led to a simple intervention.

Instead of calling patients strictly by appointment time, the clinic introduced a visible queue system. Patients could see their position in the queue and receive approximate waiting times.

At the same time, reception staff were trained to provide periodic updates.

Within a few weeks, complaints reduced significantly—not because waiting time had drastically decreased, but because uncertainty had been reduced.

This highlights an important principle: Patients are more comfortable waiting when they understand the process.

Balancing Efficiency with Human Interaction

Time management is often interpreted as speed—seeing more patients in less time. However, true efficiency in healthcare is not just about volume. It is about value per interaction.

A rushed consultation that leads to confusion may result in repeat visits, additional queries, and dissatisfaction. A slightly more attentive consultation may prevent these downstream issues.

Consider Dr. Shalini Gupta, who consciously allocates a few seconds at the beginning of each consultation to acknowledge the patient and at the end to confirm understanding. Her consultations are not significantly longer, but they are more effective.

Patients leave with clarity, reducing the need for repeated visits or follow-up calls.

Efficiency, therefore, is not compromised by respect. It is enhanced by it.

Action in Practice: Making Respect Visible in Time Management

Respect for time is not only about minimizing delays. It is about how time is experienced by the patient.

This can be achieved through simple, consistent practices.

Acknowledging delays as soon as they occur prevents frustration from building. Providing approximate waiting times creates predictability. Offering updates at regular intervals reassures patients that they have not been forgotten.

Even small gestures—such as checking in with patients who have been waiting longer—can make a significant difference.

For example, a staff member walking through the waiting area and saying, *"We appreciate your patience. The doctor will be with you shortly,"* can ease tension across the room.

A Culture of Respectful Time Management

Ultimately, time management in healthcare is not just an operational issue. It is a cultural one.

When teams begin to see waiting patients not as passive recipients but as individuals experiencing uncertainty, their approach changes.

Receptionists become communicators, not just coordinators. Nurses become guides, not just task performers. Doctors become aware not only of their schedules, but of the waiting experience they create.

This cultural shift does not require major structural changes. It requires consistent awareness and reinforcement.

Closing Reflection

Delays in healthcare are often unavoidable. Disrespect is not.

Patients understand that emergencies happen, that consultations vary, and that systems are complex. What they find difficult to accept is silence, indifference, and lack of acknowledgment.

Time, in healthcare, is more than a schedule. It is an experience.

When that experience is managed with clarity and respect, even delays can be accepted with patience.

But when it is handled poorly, even a short wait can feel long and frustrating.

The choice lies not in whether delays occur, but in how they are handled.

And in that choice, the true measure of professionalism is revealed.

Chapter 7:
The Art of Listening

Hearing What Is Said—and What Is Not

In medicine, the ability to listen is often assumed rather than taught. Questions are asked, answers are recorded, diagnoses are made. On the surface, it appears that listening is already happening.

But there is a difference between hearing words and understanding a person.

Patients rarely come with neatly structured information. They arrive with fragments—symptoms, fears, interpretations, and sometimes confusion. Within those fragments lies the truth that the clinician must uncover. The quality of that discovery depends not only on what is asked, but on how well the patient is allowed to speak.

Listening, in its true sense, is not passive. It is an active, disciplined skill. It requires attention, patience, and the ability to suspend assumptions long enough for the patient's story to unfold.

This chapter focuses on developing that discipline—so that listening becomes not an incidental part of consultation, but its foundation.

The Illusion of Listening

In a typical consultation, a pattern often emerges.

The patient begins to speak. Within a few seconds, the clinician identifies a likely direction and begins to guide the conversation. Questions become more specific, the pace quickens, and the interaction moves toward diagnosis.

This approach is efficient—but not always effective.

Consider Mr. Raghavan, a 55-year-old man who visits a clinic with complaints of dizziness. As he begins to explain, the doctor interrupts within the first few seconds and asks, *"Is it when you stand up?"*

Mr. Raghavan says yes, and the consultation proceeds along that line. Medication is prescribed accordingly.

However, what remains unexplored is that the dizziness also occurs at night, accompanied by brief episodes of blurred vision—details that could have altered the diagnostic approach.

The doctor did not ignore the patient. He simply listened selectively, guided by early assumptions.

This is the illusion of listening—where the presence of interaction creates the impression of understanding, but the depth of listening is limited.

What Active Listening Really Means

Active listening is not about staying silent. It is about being fully engaged with what the patient is saying—verbally and non-verbally—and responding in a way that encourages clarity.

It begins with giving the patient uninterrupted space to express the primary concern. This initial phase is critical. Studies and practical observations consistently show that most patients complete their initial explanation within a short span—often less than a minute—if not interrupted.

During this time, the role of the clinician is not to diagnose, but to receive.

Let us consider Mrs. Devika Nair, who comes with complaints of persistent fatigue. As she begins to speak, the doctor resists the urge to interrupt. He listens as she describes her daily routine, her sleep pattern, and her recent stress at work.

Only after she completes her explanation does he begin to ask focused questions.

By allowing her to complete her narrative, the doctor gains a more comprehensive understanding—not only of the symptom, but of the context.

Active listening also involves subtle cues that signal attention. A slight nod, a brief verbal acknowledgment such as *"I see"* or *"go on,"* and appropriate eye contact all reinforce that the patient is being heard.

These cues are small, but they create a sense of safety. Patients become more open, more detailed, and more cooperative.

Listening Beyond Words

Patients do not always express everything directly. Sometimes, what is left unsaid carries as much meaning as what is spoken.

A patient who avoids eye contact while discussing a symptom may be hesitant or embarrassed. A caregiver who repeatedly asks about a test result may be more anxious than they appear. A patient who speaks very little may be overwhelmed rather than indifferent.

Consider Anil, a young man who visits a clinic for recurring headaches. He answers questions briefly and avoids elaboration. The doctor, assuming that the issue is straightforward, proceeds with a standard line of questioning.

However, a more attentive approach reveals something else.

The doctor pauses and says, *"You seem a bit concerned. Is there something specific worrying you about these headaches?"*

Anil hesitates, then admits that he fears it might be something serious because a relative had a similar symptom before a major diagnosis.

This concern would have remained hidden without attentive listening.

Listening, therefore, is not limited to words. It includes observing tone, pace, hesitation, and emotional cues.

Interruptions: The Most Common Barrier

Interruptions are often unintentional. They arise from habit, time pressure, or the desire to guide the conversation efficiently. However, their impact is significant.

When a patient is interrupted, two things happen. First, the flow of information is disrupted. Second, the patient may feel that their input is not valued.

Let us revisit a familiar situation.

Lakshmi, a middle-aged woman, begins to describe her symptoms: *"For the past few weeks, I've been feeling a kind of heaviness in my chest, especially when—"*

The doctor interrupts, *"Is it after food?"*

Lakshmi nods, but her original sentence remains incomplete. What she intended to say was that the heaviness occurs during emotional stress, not after meals.

The interruption redirects the conversation prematurely.

Now imagine the same interaction without interruption.

Lakshmi completes her sentence, providing a clearer picture of her condition. The doctor then asks targeted questions, building on the full context.

The difference lies not in the questions asked, but in the timing of those questions.

Assumptions: The Silent Risk in Clinical Conversations

Assumptions often follow interruptions. Once an initial hypothesis is formed, the mind begins to filter information in a way that supports that hypothesis.

This is a natural cognitive process, but in clinical settings, it must be managed carefully.

Consider Dr. Karan, who sees a patient with complaints of fatigue and weight loss. Based on initial information, he assumes a lifestyle-related cause. His questions and interpretation follow that line.

However, further listening would have revealed additional symptoms pointing toward a different diagnosis.

Assumptions are not inherently wrong. They are necessary for clinical reasoning. The risk arises when they are formed too early and not revisited.

Active listening acts as a safeguard. It ensures that the initial assumption is tested against the full narrative, not just a fragment.

A Practical Shift: Structuring the Listening Process

To make listening effective in busy clinical environments, it must be structured without becoming rigid.

A simple approach can be followed in every consultation.

The first phase is uninterrupted listening, where the patient is allowed to present the primary concern.

The second phase is clarification, where the clinician

asks focused questions. The third phase is confirmation, where the clinician summarizes the understanding and checks for accuracy.

Let us see this in practice.

Patient: *"I've been having this discomfort in my stomach for a few days…"*

(Doctor listens without interruption)

Doctor: *"Alright, let me understand this better. When does it usually happen?"*

(Clarification)

After gathering information, the doctor says, *"So, you've been experiencing discomfort mainly after meals for the past week, along with some nausea. Is that correct?"*

(Confirmation)

This final step ensures that both the patient and the clinician are aligned.

Action in Practice: Training Listening as a Skill

Listening improves with deliberate practice.

In training sessions, participants can be paired and asked to simulate consultations. One person plays the patient, the other the clinician. The clinician's task is to listen without interruption for the first minute.

After the exercise, the *"patient"* shares how the interaction felt. Most often, they report feeling more comfortable and more willing to share details.

Another exercise involves identifying interruptions. Recorded or simulated consultations can be reviewed to observe where and why interruptions occur. This creates awareness of unconscious habits.

Over time, these practices help professionals develop a more disciplined approach to listening.

The Impact of Listening on Outcomes

When patients feel heard, several positive outcomes follow naturally.

They are more likely to trust the diagnosis. They are more likely to follow treatment plans. They are less likely to seek multiple opinions out of uncertainty.

From a clinical perspective, better listening leads to more accurate information, reducing the risk of misdiagnosis or incomplete assessment.

From a relational perspective, it strengthens the bond between patient and provider.

Closing Reflection

Listening is one of the simplest skills in healthcare—and one of the most powerful.

It does not require additional equipment, extended time, or complex training. It requires attention, discipline, and the willingness to pause before responding.

In a system that often prioritizes speed, listening introduces depth.

It allows the patient's story to emerge fully. It reduces assumptions. It builds trust.

And in that space—where the patient feels truly heard—healing begins, even before treatment is prescribed.

Chapter 8:
Speaking with Sensitivity

When Words Heal—and When They Harm

In healthcare, words are used constantly. Instructions are given, diagnoses are explained, updates are shared. Yet, the true impact of communication is not determined by the words alone. It is shaped by how those words are delivered, understood, and emotionally received.

A clinically correct statement can still create fear. A simple explanation, delivered with care, can create reassurance even in difficult situations.

Speaking with sensitivity is not about being overly cautious or avoiding truth. It is about delivering truth in a way that the patient can receive, understand, and process without unnecessary distress.

This chapter focuses on two critical aspects of sensitive communication: the relationship between tone and words, and the importance of avoiding medical jargon in patient interactions.

Tone vs Words: The Hidden Layer of Communication

Words carry information. Tone carries intention.

In healthcare, patients often remember the tone long after they forget the exact words. A neutral statement spoken with impatience can feel harsh. A difficult truth spoken with calmness and empathy can feel manageable.

Let us consider Mr. Daniel Fernandes, who comes in for a follow-up after a series of tests. The doctor reviews the reports and says, *"Your condition is serious. You need to start treatment immediately."*

The statement is accurate. But the tone is abrupt, direct, and without preparation.

Mr. Fernandes hears only one word: *serious*. His mind begins to race. He leaves the room anxious, confused, and overwhelmed.

Now consider the same information delivered differently.

The doctor pauses, looks at him, and says, "*I've gone through your reports. There are some concerns we need to address, but the good news is we've identified it early. Let me explain what this means and how we can manage it.*"

The diagnosis has not changed. The treatment plan remains the same.

But the patient's experience is entirely different.

The second approach prepares the patient emotionally, provides context, and introduces a sense of direction. It replaces fear with understanding.

Tone is not about being soft or vague. It is about being steady, respectful, and intentional, especially when conveying serious information.

The Emotional Impact of Everyday Language

Not all communication in healthcare involves major diagnoses. Even routine interactions carry emotional weight.

Consider Rekha, who visits a clinic for recurring headaches. After a brief consultation, the doctor says, "It's nothing. Just stress."

The intention is to reassure. But the phrase *"it's nothing*" dismisses her experience. She leaves feeling unheard and uncertain.

Now imagine the doctor saying, *“From what I see, this doesn’t appear to be serious. It’s likely related to stress, which is quite common. Let’s work on managing it so you feel better.”*
The message remains reassuring, but the patient’s concern is acknowledged rather than dismissed. Sensitive communication requires awareness of how phrases are interpreted, not just how they are intended.

Avoiding Medical Jargon: Bridging the Understanding Gap

Medical language is precise, efficient, and necessary among professionals. However, when used with patients, it often creates confusion rather than clarity.
Patients may nod in agreement, not because they understand, but because they feel uncomfortable asking for clarification.
Let us consider Ramesh, a daily wage worker diagnosed with hypertension. The doctor explains, *“You have elevated blood pressure, possibly due to lifestyle factors. You need to monitor it regularly and adhere to antihypertensive therapy.”*
Ramesh nods, collects the prescription, and leaves.
At home, he tells his family, *“The doctor said something about pressure. I think it’s okay now.”*
Two weeks later, his condition remains uncontrolled.
Now imagine the explanation given differently.
“Your blood pressure is higher than normal. This can affect your health over time if we don’t control it. You will need to take this medicine every day, even if you feel fine. We will also check it regularly.”
The second explanation is not less accurate. It is more accessible.

Avoiding jargon does not mean oversimplifying to the point of losing meaning. It means translating medical terms into language that the patient can understand and act upon.

A Real-World Scenario: When Language Creates Fear

Mrs. Shobha Iyer undergoes a diagnostic test. When she returns for the report, the technician says, *"There is a lesion. You should consult your doctor."*

The word *"lesion"* is medically correct. But for Mrs. Iyer, it is unfamiliar and alarming. She leaves the center distressed, imagining worst-case scenarios.

By the time she meets the doctor, her anxiety has escalated significantly.

Now consider an alternative approach.

"There is a small area in the report that the doctor will need to review. It's important to discuss this with them so they can guide you on the next steps."

The second explanation avoids unnecessary terminology while maintaining accuracy. It provides direction without triggering fear.

Balancing Honesty with Sensitivity

One of the most challenging aspects of communication in healthcare is balancing honesty with sensitivity.

Patients have a right to know their condition. At the same time, the way information is delivered must consider their emotional readiness.

Consider Arjun, a young professional awaiting test results. The doctor, pressed for time, says, *"It's a chronic condition. You'll have to live with it."*

The statement is truthful. But it is incomplete and emotionally abrupt.

Now imagine the same message delivered with sensitivity.

"This is a long-term condition, which means we will need to manage it over time. The good news is that with the right treatment and lifestyle changes, you can continue to live a normal and active life."

The second approach maintains honesty while providing reassurance and direction.

Sensitive communication does not dilute truth. It frames truth in a way that supports the patient's ability to cope.

Action Plan: Making Sensitive Communication a Daily Practice

Speaking with sensitivity is not an innate trait. It is a skill that can be developed through awareness and practice.

Every interaction can be approached with a simple internal check.

Before speaking, consider how the patient might receive the information. Is the tone calm and respectful? Are the words clear and understandable? Is the message complete?

During the conversation, observe the patient's response. Are they confused, anxious, or hesitant? Adjust the explanation accordingly.

After speaking, confirm understanding. A simple question such as, *"Would you like me to explain that again?"* or *"Does this make sense?"* can prevent miscommunication.

Over time, these small adjustments become natural.

A Training Exercise: Reframing Language

In training sessions, participants can be given common medical statements and asked to reframe them in patient-friendly language.

For example:

"Your condition is benign."

can become

"This is not something serious or harmful."

"You need to undergo further investigation."

can become

"We need to do a few more tests to understand this better."

Such exercises help professionals become aware of how language can be adapted without losing accuracy.

The Ripple Effect of Sensitive Communication

When patients feel understood and respected, the benefits extend beyond the immediate interaction.

They are more likely to follow instructions correctly. They are less anxious. They are more cooperative during treatment. They are more likely to return for follow-ups and recommend the facility to others.

Sensitive communication also reduces misunderstandings, repeated queries, and potential conflicts.

In this way, it improves not only patient experience, but also overall efficiency.

Closing Reflection

Words are among the most powerful tools in healthcare. They can reassure or alarm, clarify or confuse, connect or distance.

The difference lies not in complexity, but in intention.

When professionals choose words carefully, regulate their tone, and speak with awareness of the patient's emotional state, communication becomes more than an exchange of information.
It becomes a form of care.
And in that moment, healing begins—not just through treatment, but through understanding.

Chapter 9: Delivering Difficult News

When Truth Must Be Spoken with Care

There are moments in medical practice that test not clinical knowledge, but human depth. Delivering difficult news is one of them.

In such moments, patients are not simply receiving information—they are absorbing a life-altering reality. The way this reality is communicated will shape not only their understanding of the condition, but also their emotional response, their trust in the healthcare system, and their willingness to engage in treatment.

A diagnosis can be accurate and timely, yet if delivered without care, it can create shock, denial, or even disengagement. On the other hand, the same diagnosis, communicated with sensitivity and structure, can help patients process, accept, and move forward with clarity.

This chapter focuses on how to deliver difficult news in a way that is both honest and humane—ensuring that truth is not diluted, but is delivered in a manner that patients can receive and cope with.

How Difficult News is Often Delivered—And Why It Fails

In busy clinical environments, difficult conversations are sometimes handled with brevity. The intention is often efficiency or even avoidance of emotional discomfort.

Consider the following scenario.

Mr. Rajesh Kumar, a 52-year-old businessman, visits the doctor with his wife after undergoing a series of tests. He is anxious but hopeful.
The doctor reviews the reports and says, without pause, *"It's cancer. You need to start treatment immediately."*
Silence fills the room.
Mr. Kumar looks at his wife, then back at the doctor. His mind is no longer processing information. The word *cancer* echoes, overwhelming everything else.
His wife begins to ask questions, but her voice trembles. The doctor, already moving to the next point, explains treatment options in technical terms.
The consultation ends quickly.
They leave the room with more fear than clarity. This approach fails not because the information is incorrect, but because it is delivered without preparation, without emotional support, and without space for processing.
In such cases, patients often remember only the shock—not the guidance that followed.

Understanding the Patient's Psychological Moment

Before learning how to deliver difficult news, it is important to understand what the patient experiences in that moment.
When a serious diagnosis is revealed, the mind does not process information linearly. It reacts emotionally first—shock, fear, denial, confusion. Cognitive processing becomes secondary.
This means that if too much information is delivered at once, most of it will not be retained.
Consider Mrs. Latha Iyer, who receives unexpected news about a chronic condition. During the

consultation, the doctor explains the diagnosis, treatment plan, possible side effects, and follow-up schedule—all within a few minutes.

Later, when asked by her family what the doctor said, she replies, *"I don't remember everything... something about long-term treatment."*

The issue here is not comprehension. It is emotional overload.

Effective communication in such moments requires pacing, clarity, and empathy.

A Structured Approach: Simplifying the SPIKES Model

To support healthcare professionals in these conversations, a structured approach is essential. One widely used framework is the SPIKES model. However, in real-world practice, it must be adapted into a simple, practical flow that can be applied even in time-constrained settings.

Let us walk through this adapted approach step by step, using the earlier scenario.

Step 1: Setting the Environment

Before delivering the news, attention must be given to the setting.

A rushed, public, or distracted environment increases anxiety. Even in a busy hospital, small adjustments can create a more appropriate space—closing the door, sitting down, minimizing interruptions.

In Mr. Kumar's case, instead of speaking while standing or multitasking, the doctor could begin by ensuring a moment of focus.

"Mr. Kumar, please have a seat. I'd like to discuss your reports with you."

This signals that the conversation is important and deserves attention.

Step 2: Assessing What the Patient Already Knows

Patients often come with their own understanding, assumptions, or fears. Before delivering new information, it is important to understand their current perspective.

The doctor might ask,

"What have you been told so far about your tests?"

Or

"What are your thoughts about what might be causing these symptoms?"

This allows the clinician to gauge the patient's level of awareness and tailor the conversation accordingly. In some cases, patients may already suspect the seriousness. In others, they may be completely unprepared.

Step 3: Preparing the Patient for the News

Difficult news should not come abruptly. A brief preparatory statement helps the patient brace emotionally.

"I've reviewed your reports, and there are some findings that we need to discuss carefully."

This creates a transition. It signals that the information is serious without causing immediate shock.

Step 4: Delivering the Information Clearly and Gently

When the diagnosis is shared, it must be done in clear, simple language, without unnecessary technical terms, and in manageable segments.

Instead of saying,
"It's cancer. Start treatment immediately," the doctor might say,
"The reports show that there is a growth, and it has been identified as cancer."
Pause.
Allow the words to settle.
Then continue, *"I know this is difficult to hear. But the important thing is that we have identified it, and there are treatment options available."*
This approach combines clarity with compassion. It does not delay the truth, but it delivers it in a way that the patient can begin to process.

Step 5: Responding to Emotions

After the news is delivered, silence is not a gap—it is a necessary space.
Patients may react in different ways. Some may ask questions immediately. Others may remain silent. Some may express fear or disbelief.
The role of the clinician at this stage is not to move forward quickly, but to acknowledge and support the emotional response.
If Mr. Kumar looks stunned, the doctor might say, *"I can see this is a lot to take in. Please take your time."*
If his wife begins to cry, a simple, *"I understand this is very difficult,"* can provide emotional validation.
This step is often skipped, but it is critical. Without it, patients feel alone in their reaction.

Step 6: Explaining the Next Steps

Once the initial emotional response has been acknowledged, the conversation can move toward action.

At this stage, information must be given in clear, manageable parts.

"We will need to start treatment, and I will guide you through each step. The first step is to meet our oncology team, who will explain the treatment options in detail."

Avoid overwhelming the patient with too many details at once. Focus on immediate next steps.

This provides direction and reduces the sense of helplessness.

Step 7: Checking Understanding and Offering Support

Before concluding, it is important to ensure that the patient has understood the key points.

"Would you like me to go over anything again?"

"Do you have any questions right now?"

In many cases, patients may not be ready to ask questions immediately. It is helpful to reassure them that they can return with questions later.

"You don't have to remember everything today. We will go through this step by step."

This reduces pressure and builds trust.

Putting It All Together: The Improved Approach

Let us revisit the original scenario, now with the structured approach applied.

Mr. Kumar and his wife are seated. The doctor ensures privacy and begins:

"I'd like to discuss your reports with you. Before I do that, can you tell me what you've been told so far?"

After listening, the doctor continues:

"I've reviewed the reports, and there are some findings we need to talk about carefully."

Pause.

"The tests show that there is a growth, and it has been identified as cancer."
Silence.
"I know this is difficult to hear. Please take a moment."
After acknowledging their reaction, the doctor continues:
"The important thing is that we have identified it, and there are treatment options available. We will guide you through this step by step."
The conversation then moves to the next steps, with opportunities for questions and clarification.
The difference between the two approaches is not in the diagnosis. It is in the experience of receiving it.

Action Plan: Building Skill Through Practice
Delivering difficult news is not a skill that develops automatically. It requires conscious practice.
Healthcare teams can benefit from simulated role plays where participants practice these conversations in a safe environment. Feedback can focus on tone, pacing, and emotional responsiveness rather than just content.
Another useful practice is reflection. After a difficult conversation, professionals can ask themselves:

- ✓ *Did I prepare the patient before delivering the news?*
- ✓ *Did I allow space for their reaction?*
- ✓ *Did I provide clear next steps?*

Over time, this reflection strengthens awareness and improves performance.

Closing Perspective
Difficult news is part of medical reality. It cannot be avoided. But the way it is delivered can either

deepen distress or provide a pathway toward acceptance and action.

Patients may forget the exact words used. But they will always remember how they felt in that moment.

When truth is delivered with care, it does more than inform. It supports. It steadies. It builds trust at a time when trust is most needed.

And in that moment, the role of the healthcare professional extends beyond diagnosis and treatment.

It becomes an act of humanity.

Chapter 10:
Handling Caregivers with Respect

Working with the Emotions Behind the Patient

In every hospital corridor, beside almost every patient, stands someone else—watchful, anxious, and deeply invested. This person may not be the one receiving treatment, but in many ways, they are carrying an equal, if not greater, emotional burden.

They are the caregivers.

They are the son waiting outside the ICU, the wife holding a file of reports, the daughter asking questions at the nursing station, the friend managing logistics. They are the bridge between the patient and the world beyond the hospital walls.

Yet, in many healthcare interactions, caregivers are treated as secondary—sometimes even as interruptions.

This chapter addresses a critical truth: caregivers are not bystanders; they are active participants in the healing journey. How they are treated directly influences the patient's experience, the flow of care, and the overall environment within the healthcare setting.

Understanding the Emotional State of Caregivers

Caregivers rarely arrive in a calm, neutral state. They are often emotionally charged, even when they appear composed.

Their anxiety comes from multiple sources. They are worried about the patient's condition. They are responsible for making decisions, often without full understanding. They are managing time, finances, and family expectations. In many cases, they are also dealing with fatigue and lack of sleep.

Let us consider Rohit, a 32-year-old software engineer whose father has been admitted for a cardiac condition. Rohit has been at the hospital for two days, coordinating tests, speaking to relatives, and trying to understand medical updates.

By the third day, when he approaches the nurse for information and is told, *"Doctor will come and explain,"* his frustration rises quickly.

From the nurse's perspective, this is a routine response. From Rohit's perspective, it feels like avoidance. His anxiety is not just about the medical condition. It is about the lack of clarity and control.

This is the starting point for understanding caregivers. Their questions, their tone, and even their impatience are often expressions of underlying fear.

When Anxiety Turns into Friction

Caregivers under stress may ask repeated questions, seek constant updates, or appear demanding. In high-pressure environments, this can be perceived as disruptive.

Consider Mrs. Farah Khan, whose husband is in the ICU. She approaches the doctor multiple times a day, asking for updates.

- ✓ *"Is he improving?"*
- ✓ *"Why is the medication changed?"*
- ✓ *"When will he be shifted?"*

By the third interaction, the doctor, already managing multiple critical cases, responds briefly, *"We are doing what is necessary. Please wait."*

Mrs. Khan feels dismissed. Her anxiety increases. She begins to interpret the lack of detailed response as a sign that something is being hidden.

A cycle begins—her questions increase, the responses become shorter, and the tension escalates.

This situation is common, and it highlights an important principle: When anxiety is not addressed, it often turns into friction.

Reframing the Caregiver's Role

To manage caregivers effectively, there must be a shift in perception.

Caregivers are not obstacles to efficiency. They are partners in care.

They are the ones who will ensure that medications are taken correctly after discharge. They will observe symptoms at home, manage follow-ups, and provide emotional support to the patient.

When caregivers are informed and reassured, they become allies. When they are confused or ignored, they become anxious—and sometimes confrontational.

Let us look at a different approach.

Scenario: Two Ways of Handling the Same Caregiver

Situation: A patient is undergoing treatment, and the caregiver approaches for an update.

Approach One

Caregiver: *"Doctor, can you tell me how my father is doing?"*

Doctor (while walking): *"We will update you later."*

The caregiver is left uncertain. The response is brief, but it creates emotional distance.

Approach Two

Caregiver: *"Doctor, can you tell me how my father is doing?"*

Doctor (pauses briefly): *"He is stable at the moment. We are monitoring him closely. I will be able to give you a more detailed update in about an hour."*

The second response takes only a few seconds longer, but it provides reassurance, clarity, and a timeline.

The difference lies not in the information, but in the engagement.

Managing Questions: From Repetition to Reassurance

One of the most common challenges with caregivers is repeated questioning.

At first glance, this may seem inefficient. However, repeated questions are often a sign that the caregiver has not fully understood or felt reassured by previous responses.

Consider Anita, whose mother is undergoing treatment. She asks the nurse multiple times, *"When will the reports come?"* Each time, she receives the same answer: *"By evening."*

By afternoon, she asks again—not because she forgot, but because she is anxious.

Now imagine a different response.

"It should be ready by evening, around 5 p.m. I understand you're waiting for it. As soon as it comes, we will inform you immediately."

The added context and acknowledgment reduce the need for repeated questioning.

Managing questions is not about limiting them. It is about addressing the underlying concern clearly and completely.

Providing Structure to Reduce Anxiety

Uncertainty is one of the biggest sources of stress for caregivers. When they do not know what will happen next, their anxiety increases.

Providing structure can significantly reduce this.

Let us consider Mr. Subramanian, whose wife has been admitted for observation. He is unsure about the process—when the doctor will visit, when tests will be done, and how long the stay will be.

If left uninformed, he will seek answers repeatedly.

Now imagine that at the time of admission, a staff member explains:

"The doctor will visit twice a day—once in the morning and once in the evening. Tests are usually done before noon, and reports come by evening. If there are any changes, we will inform you immediately."

This simple orientation provides a framework. It reduces uncertainty and, with it, anxiety.

Caregivers do not expect constant updates. They expect predictability.

Balancing Boundaries with Accessibility

While it is important to engage with caregivers, boundaries must also be maintained. Healthcare professionals cannot be available at all times for extended discussions.

The key is to balance accessibility with structure.

Instead of responding to repeated interruptions, a more effective approach is to create designated communication points.

For example, a doctor might say:

"I will be available to speak with you after the evening rounds. At that time, I can give you a detailed update."

This sets a clear expectation and reduces unscheduled interruptions.

At the same time, caregivers must feel that they have a channel for urgent concerns.

"If there is anything urgent, please inform the nurse, and I will be notified."

This balance ensures that caregivers feel supported without overwhelming the system.

Action in Practice: Building Respectful Caregiver Interactions

Handling caregivers with respect requires consistency in small actions.

Acknowledging their presence, even briefly, makes a difference. Explaining delays or changes in plans reduces frustration. Providing clear timelines helps manage expectations.

In training environments, staff can be encouraged to view every caregiver interaction through a simple lens:

"What is this person feeling right now, and what do they need to feel more at ease?"

This question shifts the focus from task completion to human engagement.

A Training Exercise: Walking in the Caregiver's Shoes

One effective way to build empathy is through simulation.

Participants can be asked to role-play as caregivers in a hospital setting. They are given a scenario—waiting for a test result, seeking an update, or managing a sudden change in condition.

Another group plays the role of healthcare staff.

After the exercise, caregivers share their experience. Most often, they describe feelings of uncertainty, anxiety, and the need for reassurance.
This exercise creates immediate awareness of how small interactions impact emotional experience.

The Ripple Effect of Respectful Engagement

When caregivers are treated with respect, the benefits extend beyond the interaction.
They become calmer and more cooperative. They communicate more effectively with the patient. They are better prepared to manage care after discharge.
From the perspective of the healthcare team, this reduces repeated interruptions, misunderstandings, and potential conflicts.
Respect, therefore, is not just a value. It is a practical tool for improving efficiency and outcomes.

Closing Reflection

Behind every patient is a caregiver carrying unseen weight.
They may not wear a hospital badge. They may not have medical training. But they are deeply involved in the journey.
When they are ignored, the environment becomes tense. When they are respected, the environment becomes supportive.
Handling caregivers with respect is not about giving them more time. It is about giving them clarity, acknowledgment, and reassurance.
In doing so, healthcare professionals do more than manage interactions.
They create an atmosphere where care is not confined to the patient alone—but extends to everyone who stands beside them.

And in that environment, healing becomes a shared experience.

Chapter 11:
Front Desk is the Frontline

Where Patient Experience Truly Begins

Long before a doctor speaks, before a diagnosis is made, before any treatment begins, a patient has already formed an impression of the healthcare facility.

That impression is shaped at the front desk.

It is here that anxiety meets response. It is here that confusion meets clarity—or sometimes, indifference. It is here that the tone of the entire experience is set.

Hospitals often invest heavily in clinical excellence, infrastructure, and technology. Yet, the most powerful determinant of patient perception is often a brief interaction at the reception counter.

This chapter brings into focus a simple but often overlooked truth: the front desk is not an administrative function—it is the frontline of patient experience.

The First Impression: Formed in Seconds, Lasting for Years

Patients rarely arrive in a relaxed state. Even for routine visits, there is some level of concern. For more serious conditions, anxiety is already high before they step through the door.

Now consider what happens next.

Mr. Sandeep Pillai, visiting a hospital for the first time, approaches the reception counter. He is unsure where to go, what to do, and how long the process will take.

He says, *"I have an appointment with Dr. Kumar."*

The receptionist, without looking up, responds, "*Token. Sit.*"

Mr. Pillai steps aside, unsure of what just happened. He looks around, trying to understand the process.

In that moment, the hospital has already communicated something—not through policy or branding, but through behavior.

Now imagine the same situation handled differently.

The receptionist looks up, makes brief eye contact, and says, *"Good morning. You have an appointment with Dr. Kumar? Let me guide you. Please take this token and have a seat. The doctor is currently seeing patients, and your turn should come in about 20 minutes."*

The difference is not in the system. It is in the delivery of the system.

First impressions are not formed by complexity. They are formed by clarity, tone, and attention.

The Front Desk as an Emotional Filter

The reception area acts as a filter through which patient emotions either settle or escalate.

A patient who is anxious can be reassured in a few seconds with the right response. The same patient can become more anxious if met with indifference.

Let us consider Mrs. Kavya Reddy, who arrives with her elderly mother for a consultation. Her mother is visibly uncomfortable, and Kavya is trying to manage both the situation and the process.

At the reception, she asks, *"Where do we go for the consultation?"*

If the response is, "*Go there,*" accompanied by a vague gesture, her stress increases. She must now navigate an unfamiliar system while caring for her mother.

If the response is, *"Let me show you. Please go to the second floor, room 204. If you need help, there is a staff member near the lift,"* the experience changes.

The front desk does not just manage information. It manages emotional flow.

Why Reception Staff Are Often Underestimated

In many healthcare settings, reception roles are seen as entry-level administrative positions. Training is focused on process—registration, billing, scheduling—while the human aspect of the role is left to individual personality.

This is a critical gap.

Reception staff interact with every patient. They handle first-time visitors, repeat patients, anxious caregivers, and sometimes even distressed families. They are required to manage volume, maintain accuracy, and respond quickly.

Without proper training, they fall back on efficiency alone—short responses, minimal engagement, and task-focused behavior.

This is not a failure of intention. It is a failure of preparation.

To transform patient experience, the front desk must be recognized and trained as a patient-facing role of strategic importance.

A Real-World Scenario: When Process Overrides Experience

Ravi, a young man visiting for a diagnostic test, approaches the reception.

"I've come for a blood test."

The receptionist, handling multiple tasks, says, *"Fill this form."*

Ravi fills the form and returns.
"Go to billing."
After billing, he asks, "*Where is the lab?*"
"Downstairs."
Each response is technically correct. Yet Ravi feels like he is navigating the system alone.
Now consider a structured approach.
When Ravi first arrives, the receptionist says, *"Welcome. You're here for a blood test? Please fill this form. After that, go to billing at counter 2, and then proceed to the lab on the ground floor. If you need help, please let me know."*
The process is the same. The experience is guided.
The difference lies in anticipating the patient's journey instead of reacting to each step.

Training Reception Staff: From Transaction to Interaction

To elevate the front desk experience, training must go beyond procedural instructions. It must focus on communication, empathy, and clarity.
Reception staff must be trained to recognize that every patient interaction carries emotional weight. A simple question may carry anxiety. A request for information may reflect uncertainty.
Training should include real-life scenarios where staff practice responding to different types of patients—first-time visitors, elderly individuals, anxious caregivers, and even frustrated patients.
For example, a staff member can be trained to respond to a delayed appointment not with *"Doctor is late,"* but with, "*The doctor is delayed due to an emergency. We expect a wait of about 30 minutes. Thank you for your patience.*"

This shift requires awareness, practice, and reinforcement.

Building Consistency Across the Front Desk

One of the challenges in healthcare settings is inconsistency. One staff member may be courteous and helpful, while another may be abrupt.

From the patient's perspective, this inconsistency creates confusion about what to expect.

To address this, clear communication standards must be established.

Every patient should be greeted. Every process should be explained. Every delay should be communicated. Every query should be acknowledged.

These are not complex protocols. They are behavioral standards that define the culture of the organization.

Action in Practice: Simple Changes with Immediate Impact

Improving front desk experience does not require major investment. It requires attention to detail.

A simple greeting can set a positive tone. Clear directions can reduce confusion. A brief explanation of waiting time can reduce frustration.

Consider a clinic that introduced a small change. Reception staff were trained to provide a short orientation to every new patient—where to go, what to expect, and how long it might take.

Within weeks, patient feedback improved significantly. Not because the system changed, but because the experience of the system became clearer.

Handling Difficult Situations at the Front Desk

Reception staff often face challenging situations—patients who are upset about delays, caregivers who are anxious, or individuals who are confused.

In such moments, the instinct may be to respond quickly and move on. However, a brief moment of acknowledgment can de-escalate the situation.

For example, when a patient says, *"I've been waiting for a long time,"* the response should not be defensive.

Instead, *"I understand you've been waiting. Let me check your status and update you,"* creates a sense of being heard.

This approach does not require additional authority. It requires emotional awareness.

A Training Exercise: The First 60 Seconds

In training sessions, reception staff can be asked to simulate the first 60 seconds of a patient interaction.

One participant plays the patient, another the receptionist.

The focus is on greeting, clarity, and tone.

After the exercise, the "patient" shares how the interaction felt.

This exercise often reveals how small changes—eye contact, tone, and clear instructions—can transform the experience.

Repeated practice helps build confidence and consistency.

The Ripple Effect of a Strong Front Desk

When the front desk functions effectively, the impact extends throughout the system.

Patients arrive at consultation rooms calmer and better informed. Doctors spend less time clarifying

basic processes. Nurses receive fewer repetitive queries. Overall flow improves.
Conversely, when the front desk is weak, the entire system feels disorganized, regardless of clinical excellence.

Closing Reflection

The front desk is often the first point of contact—and sometimes the last.
It is where patients form their first impression and where they decide whether they feel confident in the system they have entered.
When handled well, it creates a sense of order, reassurance, and trust. When neglected, it creates confusion and anxiety.
The transformation does not require complex systems. It requires a shift in perspective.
Reception staff are not just managing entries and exits. They are shaping experiences.
And in that role, they are not at the periphery of healthcare.
They are at its frontline.

Chapter 12: Nursing Excellence & Patient Experience

The Human Bridge Between Treatment and Comfort

In the daily rhythm of a hospital, doctors often make the critical decisions, but it is the nurses who carry those decisions into lived experience. They are present at the bedside when pain rises, when fear surfaces, when confusion sets in, and when recovery begins. If the hospital were a journey, nurses would not merely be guides—they would be companions walking alongside the patient at every step.

For many patients, the nurse is not just a caregiver, but the most consistent human connection within the system. It is the nurse who answers the call bell at night, who adjusts a pillow, who explains a medication, who notices discomfort before it is spoken. In moments when the patient feels most vulnerable, it is often the nurse who becomes the emotional anchor.

This chapter explores the depth of that role—how nursing excellence is not only clinical precision, but emotional steadiness, and how communication during procedures can transform fear into trust.

Nurses as Emotional Anchors

Patients enter healthcare environments with varying degrees of fear. Some are anxious about a diagnosis, others about pain, others about the unknown. In such moments, clinical competence alone is not enough. Patients look for reassurance, stability, and presence.

Let us consider Mr. Joseph D'Souza, a 68-year-old patient admitted for a surgical procedure. The day before the surgery, he appears restless. He asks repeated questions, struggles to sleep, and seems withdrawn.

During the evening round, Nurse Anitha notices his unease. Instead of limiting her interaction to routine checks, she pauses and asks, *"Are you feeling worried about tomorrow?"*

Mr. D'Souza nods. He speaks slowly, expressing fear about the surgery and the outcome.

Nurse Anitha does not rush the moment. She listens. She reassures him in simple, calm language. She explains what will happen the next day in a way he can understand.

That night, Mr. D'Souza sleeps better.

Nothing about the surgery has changed. But his emotional state has.

This is the role of the nurse as an emotional anchor—not to provide all the answers, but to create a sense of safety.

The Power of Presence

In many situations, patients do not expect long conversations. They expect presence.

Presence is not measured in minutes. It is measured in attention.

A nurse who pauses, makes eye contact, and acknowledges a concern—even briefly—can create more reassurance than a longer interaction delivered without focus.

Consider Priya, a young woman admitted for observation. She presses the call bell because she feels uneasy, though she cannot clearly explain why.

The nurse arrives and says, *"Yes, what do you need?"* while adjusting equipment.

Priya hesitates. *"Nothing… I just felt uncomfortable."*

The nurse leaves quickly.

Priya feels dismissed, even though her concern was not clinical.

Now imagine a different response.

The nurse arrives, sits briefly beside her, and says, *"You seem a little uneasy. Tell me what you're feeling."*

Priya opens up about her anxiety.

The nurse listens, reassures her, and stays for a moment longer before leaving.

The difference is not in time, but in quality of attention.

Communication During Procedures: The Unseen Gap

Procedures—whether minor or major—are moments of heightened vulnerability for patients. Even a simple injection or blood draw can trigger anxiety, especially when the patient does not know what to expect.

In many healthcare settings, procedures are performed efficiently but with minimal communication.

Let us consider Rahul, a teenager undergoing a routine blood test. He sits nervously, watching the nurse prepare the equipment.

Without explanation, the nurse proceeds. Rahul flinches as the needle is inserted. His anxiety increases for future visits.

Now imagine the same procedure handled differently.

The nurse says, *"Rahul, I'm going to take a small blood sample. You will feel a quick pinch, but it will be over in a few seconds. Try to relax your arm."*

She maintains a calm tone and observes his reaction.

The procedure is completed smoothly. Rahul feels more at ease.

The difference lies in preparation and communication.

Reducing Fear Through Explanation

Patients often fear what they do not understand. A brief explanation can significantly reduce that fear.

Consider Mrs. Meenakshi Iyer, who is about to receive an intravenous line for the first time. She appears tense, holding her arm stiffly.

If the nurse proceeds without explanation, the patient's discomfort increases.

Instead, the nurse says, *"I'm going to insert a small tube into your vein so we can give you medication. You may feel a slight discomfort for a moment. Once it's in place, it should feel comfortable."*

This explanation does not eliminate the sensation, but it reduces uncertainty.

Patients who know what to expect are more cooperative and less anxious.

The Role of Tone During Procedures

During procedures, tone becomes as important as technique.

A hurried or mechanical tone can increase anxiety, even if the procedure is done perfectly. A calm and steady tone reassures the patient.

Let us consider Mr. Ahmed, who requires a dressing change after surgery. The nurse approaches with efficiency, focusing on completing the task.
If the nurse says, *"This might hurt,"* in a flat or abrupt tone, the patient braces for pain.
Now imagine the nurse saying, *"You may feel some discomfort as I change the dressing. I'll go slowly, and if it becomes too uncomfortable, let me know."*
The second approach gives the patient a sense of control.
Tone, in such moments, becomes a form of care.

Building Trust Through Consistency
Patients observe patterns. When nurses consistently communicate, explain, and respond with care, trust builds naturally.
Consider a ward where nurses routinely inform patients before administering medication, explain procedures briefly, and check for comfort afterward.
Patients in such an environment feel more secure. They are less likely to resist procedures, less anxious, and more cooperative.
Consistency transforms individual acts of care into a culture of care.

A Practical Scenario: The Difference in Experience
Scenario One
A nurse enters, administers an injection without explanation, and leaves.
The patient feels startled, unsure of what was given, and slightly anxious.
Scenario Two

A nurse enters and says, *"I'm going to give you your medication now. It's an injection that will help reduce your pain. You may feel a slight sting."*
After administering, she adds, *"How are you feeling? Is it comfortable?"*
The patient feels informed and reassured.
The clinical act is identical. The experience is not.

Action in Practice: Making Nursing Excellence Visible

Nursing excellence must be made visible through everyday actions.
Before any procedure, a brief explanation should be given. During the procedure, the patient's comfort should be observed. After the procedure, reassurance should be provided.
These steps do not add significant time. They add value.
Hospitals can incorporate these practices into standard protocols—not as rigid scripts, but as guiding principles.
Training sessions can include role plays where nurses practice explaining procedures in simple language, adjusting tone, and responding to patient reactions.

A Training Exercise: The Silent Procedure vs The Explained Procedure

In a training setting, participants can be asked to perform a simulated procedure in two ways.
In the first round, the procedure is done without any communication.
In the second round, the procedure is explained before, during, and after.

Participants playing the role of patients are then asked to describe their experience.
The contrast is often striking.
This exercise reinforces a powerful lesson: Communication is not an addition to care—it is part of care.

Supporting Nurses in Their Role

It is important to recognize that nurses operate under significant pressure. High patient loads, long shifts, and administrative demands can make it challenging to maintain consistent communication.
For nursing excellence to thrive, the system must support it.
Adequate staffing, clear protocols, and a culture that values patient experience are essential. Recognition of good practice also plays a role. When nurses see that their efforts in communication and empathy are valued, they are more likely to sustain them.

Closing Reflection

Nurses stand at the intersection of treatment and experience.
They translate medical decisions into human care. They witness the patient's journey not in isolated moments, but in continuity.
When they act as emotional anchors, patients feel supported. When they communicate during procedures, patients feel informed. When they combine skill with sensitivity, patients feel safe.
In many ways, the patient's memory of a hospital is shaped not by the complexity of treatment, but by the presence of those who cared for them most consistently.
And more often than not, that presence is the nurse.

In recognizing and strengthening this role, healthcare moves closer to what it is meant to be—not just a system of treatment, but a space of healing.

Chapter 13:
Cleanliness, Environment & Dignity

The Silent Language of Care

In healthcare, much attention is given to diagnosis, treatment, and clinical outcomes. Yet, long before a patient experiences any of these, they encounter something more immediate—the environment.

The cleanliness of a corridor, the smell of a ward, the clarity of signage, the privacy of a consultation space—these are not secondary details. They are powerful signals that communicate how much a system values the people within it.

Patients may not have the expertise to evaluate clinical decisions, but they are highly perceptive of their surroundings. The environment becomes their first measure of safety, competence, and respect.

This chapter explores how cleanliness, physical space, and dignity are not peripheral concerns, but central to healing and patient experience.

The Environment as a Message

Every healthcare setting sends a message, whether intended or not.

A clean, well-organized space communicates care, discipline, and professionalism. A cluttered or poorly maintained space communicates neglect, even if the clinical care is excellent.

Let us consider Mr. Arul Prakash, who visits a hospital for a minor procedure. As he walks in, he notices the waiting area—chairs arranged neatly, floors clean, clear directions displayed.

He feels reassured, even before meeting the doctor.

Now imagine a different scenario.
He enters a facility where the floor is stained, the seating area is disorganized, and there is a lingering odor. Even before any interaction, a sense of discomfort sets in.
The treatment may be the same in both settings. But the patient's confidence is not.
The environment speaks before any human does.

Cleanliness: More Than Hygiene
Cleanliness in healthcare is often associated with infection control, and rightly so. However, its impact goes beyond clinical safety.
It influences perception, trust, and emotional comfort.
Consider Mrs. Nalini Krishnan, admitted for a short stay. Her room is clinically safe, but the bedsheet is slightly wrinkled, the dustbin is not emptied on time, and the washroom shows signs of neglect.
None of these may directly affect her treatment, but they affect her sense of being cared for.
Now imagine the same room maintained with attention—fresh linen, clean surfaces, a well-kept washroom.
Mrs. Krishnan feels more comfortable, more at ease, and more confident in the care she is receiving.
Cleanliness is not only about preventing infection. It is about creating an environment where patients feel valued.

The Role of Sensory Experience
Patients experience the environment through all their senses.
Sight, smell, sound, and even touch contribute to their perception.

A strong disinfectant smell may signal cleanliness to some, but to others, it may feel overwhelming. Loud conversations at nursing stations may seem routine to staff, but they can disturb patients trying to rest.

Consider Rahul, recovering from a procedure. He lies in bed, trying to rest, but hears continuous noise from the corridor—trolleys, conversations, announcements.

His physical recovery is not directly affected, but his comfort is.

Now imagine a quieter environment, where noise is managed, and patient rest is considered.

Healing is not only physical. It is also environmental.

Privacy: The Foundation of Dignity

Among all aspects of the environment, privacy holds a unique place. It is directly linked to dignity.

Patients often share deeply personal information—about their bodies, their conditions, their fears. They undergo examinations and procedures that leave them physically and emotionally exposed.

In such moments, privacy is not a luxury. It is a necessity.

Let us consider Ms. Aisha Begum, who visits for a consultation regarding a sensitive health issue. As she speaks, other patients and staff move around within earshot.

She lowers her voice, hesitates, and omits details.

The consultation is incomplete—not because of lack of competence, but because of lack of privacy.

Now imagine the same consultation in a space where the door is closed, interruptions are minimized, and the patient feels secure.

Ms. Begum speaks openly. The doctor receives complete information. The quality of care improves.

Privacy directly influences communication, and communication influences outcomes.

Maintaining Dignity During Care

Dignity is not only about space. It is about how patients are treated during care.

Consider Mr. Suresh, who requires assistance with mobility after surgery. If he is moved or assisted without explanation, or if his discomfort is not acknowledged, he may feel embarrassed or diminished.

Now imagine a nurse saying, *"I'm going to help you sit up. Please take your time. Let me know if you feel uncomfortable."*

This simple communication preserves dignity.

Similarly, during examinations or procedures, covering the patient appropriately, explaining steps, and seeking consent are essential.

Dignity is maintained not through grand gestures, but through consistent respect in small actions.

Signage: Guiding Without Confusion

Hospitals can be complex spaces. Multiple departments, floors, and processes can easily overwhelm a patient or caregiver.

Clear signage is often underestimated, yet it plays a critical role in reducing stress.

Let us consider Mr. Karthik, visiting for a diagnostic test. He moves from one corridor to another, unsure of where to go. He hesitates to ask for directions repeatedly.

By the time he reaches the correct location, he is already frustrated.

Now imagine a facility with clear, visible signage—directions to departments, floors clearly marked, processes explained.
Mr. Karthik navigates the space with ease.
Signage is not just about direction. It is about reducing uncertainty.

A Practical Scenario: Environment and Experience

Scenario One

A patient enters a ward where beds are unorganized, staff move hurriedly, and there is little attention to cleanliness or privacy.
Even before treatment begins, the patient feels uneasy.

Scenario Two

A patient enters a ward where everything is orderly, clean, and clearly structured. Staff move with purpose, and the environment feels calm.
The patient feels reassured.
The difference is not in clinical expertise. It is in the environmental experience.

Action in Practice: Creating a Healing Environment

Improving environment and dignity does not always require large investments. It requires attention, ownership, and consistency.
Regular checks for cleanliness, timely maintenance, and accountability for shared spaces are essential.
Staff must be trained to see the environment through the patient's eyes. A corridor is not just a passage; it is part of the patient's journey. A waiting area is not just a space; it is where anxiety builds or settles.

Simple practices—ensuring washrooms are clean, maintaining quiet zones, organizing seating, and updating signage—can have immediate impact.

A Training Exercise: The Patient Walkthrough

One effective way to build awareness is to conduct a "patient walkthrough."

Staff members are asked to walk through the facility as if they were patients—entering from the main gate, navigating to different departments, using the waiting areas, and observing the environment.

They are then asked to reflect on their experience.

- ✓ *Where did they feel confused?*
- ✓ *Where did they feel uncomfortable?*
- ✓ *What could be improved?*

This exercise often reveals gaps that are otherwise overlooked.

The Culture of Ownership

For environment and dignity to be maintained, responsibility cannot rest with one department alone.

Housekeeping ensures cleanliness, but every staff member contributes to maintaining it. Nurses ensure patient comfort, but the environment must support their efforts. Administrators design systems, but daily practice sustains them.

When everyone takes ownership, the environment reflects care.

Closing Reflection

Healing does not happen in isolation. It happens within a space.

That space can either support recovery or add to discomfort.

Cleanliness reassures. Privacy protects dignity. Clear signage reduces confusion. A well-maintained environment creates trust.

Patients may not always articulate these elements, but they feel them.

And in those feelings lies a powerful truth:

Before treatment begins, the environment has already begun to heal—or to harm.

The choice of which it does lies in the attention given to the smallest details.

And in healthcare, it is often those details that make the greatest difference.

Chapter 14: Reducing Waiting Frustration

Designing Systems That Patients Can Trust

Waiting is an unavoidable part of healthcare. Patients wait for consultations, for tests, for reports, for discharge, and sometimes for answers that take time to emerge. Yet, what patients struggle with is not waiting itself—it is uncertain waiting.

A ten-minute wait without clarity can feel longer than a thirty-minute wait with clear communication. This distinction is often misunderstood. Healthcare systems tend to focus on reducing waiting time, which is important, but equally critical is managing how waiting is experienced.

This chapter explores how a systems-thinking approach and transparent queue management can transform waiting from a source of frustration into a manageable, even acceptable, part of care.

Understanding Waiting as a System Issue

Waiting is rarely the result of a single delay. It is usually the outcome of interconnected processes.

A consultation runs longer than expected. A test report is delayed. A doctor is called into an emergency. A patient arrives late but must still be accommodated. Over time, these small variations accumulate, creating a backlog.

From within the system, these are understandable events. From outside, for the patient, it appears as inefficiency.

Let us consider Dr. Meera Nair's clinic, where appointments are scheduled every ten minutes. In reality, consultations vary widely. Some take five minutes, others take twenty. By mid-morning, the schedule is already misaligned.

Patients continue to arrive on time, but the system is running behind.

Each individual delay has a reason. But collectively, they create a pattern of waiting.

This is where systems thinking becomes essential. Instead of addressing delays individually, the focus must shift to how the entire flow operates.

The Patient's Experience of Waiting

To design better systems, one must first understand what waiting feels like from the patient's perspective.

Consider Mr. Vinod Sharma, who arrives at 9:45 a.m. for a 10:00 a.m. appointment. By 10:30, he is still waiting. There has been no update.

He begins to check the time repeatedly. He wonders if he has been forgotten. He considers approaching the reception but hesitates.

By 11:00, his frustration has grown—not only because of the delay, but because of the lack of information.

Now imagine a different experience.

At 10:05, the receptionist informs the waiting area, *"The doctor is currently running about 20 minutes behind schedule due to a longer consultation. We appreciate your patience."*

At 10:30, another update is given.

Mr. Sharma is still waiting. But he is not uncertain.

The difference lies in predictability.

Systems Thinking: Designing for Flow, Not Just Speed

Improving patient flow is not about pushing more patients through the system. It is about aligning processes so that movement is smoother and more predictable.

In many healthcare settings, scheduling is done uniformly—every patient is given the same time slot. However, not all consultations are equal.

A follow-up visit may take significantly less time than a first consultation. A complex case may require more time than anticipated.

Let us consider a clinic that introduced a simple change.

Appointments were categorized into types—new consultations, follow-ups, and review visits. Each category was given a different time allocation. Additionally, buffer slots were introduced every hour to absorb unexpected delays.

Within weeks, the overall flow improved. Waiting time did not disappear, but it became more consistent and manageable.

This is the essence of systems thinking—recognizing patterns and designing processes that accommodate variation.

Queue Transparency: Turning Uncertainty into Clarity

One of the most effective ways to reduce waiting frustration is to make the queue visible. When patients can see where they stand in the process, their perception of waiting changes.

Consider Lakshmi, waiting for her turn in a crowded outpatient department. She has no idea how many

patients are ahead of her. Every time a name is called, she wonders if hers will be next.
Now imagine a system where a display shows the current token number and the next few in line.
Lakshmi can see that there are five patients ahead of her. She has a sense of position and progression.
The waiting time has not changed. But her experience has.
Queue transparency reduces anxiety by replacing uncertainty with information.

A Practical Scenario: The Power of Visibility

Scenario One

Patients sit in a waiting area with no clear order. Names are called unpredictably. Some patients feel that others are being seen out of turn.
Frustration builds, even if the system is functioning correctly.

Scenario Two

Patients are given tokens. A display shows the current number. Staff periodically announce updates.
Even if delays occur, the process feels fair and structured.
The second scenario creates trust, even in the presence of waiting.

Communicating Delays: A System, Not an Afterthought

Communication about delays is often reactive. Patients ask, and staff respond.
A more effective approach is proactive communication.
Consider a hospital that implemented a simple protocol. Every 20–30 minutes, the reception staff

provided an update to the waiting area, even if there was no significant change.

"We are currently running about 25 minutes behind. Thank you for your patience."

This reduced the number of individual queries and created a sense of collective awareness.

Patients no longer felt the need to ask repeatedly. The system was already informing them.

Managing Expectations at the Start

One of the most overlooked opportunities to reduce frustration is at the very beginning of the patient journey.

When patients arrive, they often have an expectation of how long the process will take. If this expectation is not aligned with reality, frustration is inevitable.

Consider Mr. Harish, who arrives expecting to be seen within 15 minutes. When the wait extends to 45 minutes, he feels dissatisfied.

Now imagine if, at the time of registration, he is informed:

"The current waiting time is approximately 40–45 minutes."

His expectation is adjusted. The same waiting time now feels acceptable.

Expectation management is not about lowering standards. It is about aligning perception with reality.

Action in Practice: Designing a Patient-Friendly Waiting Experience

Reducing waiting frustration requires a combination of structure and communication.

Systems must be designed to handle variation—through categorized appointments, buffer slots, and coordinated scheduling.

At the same time, communication must be clear, consistent, and proactive.

Patients should know where they are in the process, how long they might wait, and what to expect next.

Even small additions—such as displaying queue status, providing estimated waiting times, or offering updates—can significantly improve the experience.

A Training Exercise: The Waiting Room Simulation

In training sessions, staff can be asked to experience the waiting process themselves.

Participants are given a token and asked to wait without any information. After a few minutes, they are asked to reflect on how they feel.

In the second round, the same waiting is accompanied by regular updates and visible queue status.

The difference in emotional response is immediate.

This exercise helps staff understand that waiting is not just a logistical issue—it is an emotional experience.

The Ripple Effect of Better Systems

When waiting is managed effectively, the benefits extend across the organization.

Patients are calmer and more cooperative. Staff face fewer interruptions and complaints. Doctors can focus on consultations without constant pressure from the waiting area.

A well-managed system creates a smoother flow, not only of patients, but of interactions.

Closing Reflection

Waiting cannot be eliminated from healthcare. But frustration can be.

The key lies in shifting from a focus on time alone to a focus on experience.

When systems are designed thoughtfully and communication is handled with clarity, waiting becomes predictable rather than stressful.

Patients do not expect perfection. They expect fairness, transparency, and respect.

When those are present, even a delay becomes manageable.

And in that shift—from uncertainty to clarity—the patient experience is transformed.

Chapter 15:
Handling Angry Patients

Turning Confrontation into Constructive Care

Anger is one of the most visible and challenging emotions encountered in healthcare settings. It can surface at the reception desk, in the waiting area, inside consultation rooms, or at the billing counter. It may come from patients themselves or from caregivers who are under strain.

For healthcare professionals, these moments are often uncomfortable and disruptive. The instinct may be to defend, correct, or withdraw. However, when handled poorly, anger escalates quickly—affecting not only the immediate interaction but also the environment around it.

This chapter approaches anger not as a problem to be suppressed, but as a signal to be understood and managed. Behind most anger in healthcare lies fear, uncertainty, pain, or perceived neglect. The goal is not to "win" the interaction, but to restore calm, clarity, and trust.

Understanding the Source of Anger

Anger rarely appears without cause. It is often the final expression of an unmet need.

A patient who has waited too long without updates may feel ignored. A caregiver who does not understand a diagnosis may feel helpless. A billing discrepancy may trigger a sense of unfairness. Pain, fear, and fatigue amplify these reactions.

Consider Mr. Ramesh Iyer, who has been waiting for over an hour for his appointment. No updates have been provided. When he finally approaches the desk, his voice is raised.

"What is going on here? Why am I waiting so long?"

From the staff's perspective, this may appear as impatience. From Mr. Iyer's perspective, it is frustration built over time.

If the response is defensive—*"You have to wait, there are other patients"*—the situation escalates.

If the response acknowledges his experience—*"I understand you've been waiting, and I'm sorry for the delay. Let me check your status"*—the tone begins to shift.

The first step in handling anger is recognizing that it is often an expression of distress, not disrespect.

The Escalation Pattern

Anger tends to follow a predictable pattern.

It begins with frustration. If not addressed, it grows into irritation. When still unaddressed, it becomes confrontation.

At each stage, there is an opportunity to intervene.

Consider Mrs. Sunita Kapoor, waiting for her husband's test results. Initially, she asks politely. When she receives vague answers, her tone becomes sharper. Eventually, she raises her voice at the staff.

By the time the situation reaches confrontation, it feels difficult to manage.

However, if her concern had been addressed earlier—through clear communication and reassurance—the escalation could have been prevented.

Understanding this pattern allows healthcare professionals to act early, before anger intensifies.

De-escalation: The Art of Calming the Moment

De-escalation is not about controlling the other person. It is about managing the interaction in a way that reduces intensity.

The first principle of de-escalation is not to match the emotion.

When a patient raises their voice, the natural reaction may be to respond with equal firmness. This often leads to escalation.

Instead, the response must be calm, steady, and controlled.

Let us consider a scenario.

Mr. Ahmed, frustrated with a billing issue, says loudly, *"This is completely unacceptable! You people don't know what you're doing!"*

If the staff member responds defensively, *"You need to calm down first,"* the situation worsens.

Now imagine a different response.

"I can see that this is frustrating. Let me understand what happened so I can help resolve it."

This response does three things at once. It acknowledges emotion, shifts focus to the issue, and signals willingness to help.

De-escalation begins with acknowledgment, not argument.

The Power of Listening in Heated Moments

When people are angry, they want to be heard. Interrupting or correcting them too quickly can increase their intensity.

Consider Vikram, who is upset about a delay in discharge. He begins to explain his frustration, but the staff member interrupts to justify the delay.

Vikram raises his voice further.

Now imagine the staff member allowing him to speak fully, even if his tone is strong.

After he finishes, the staff member responds, *"I understand why this is frustrating. Let me explain what is causing the delay and how we can move this forward."*

By allowing expression first, the emotional intensity reduces.

Listening, in such moments, is not passive. It is a strategic tool for calming the situation.

Staying Calm Under Pressure

Handling anger effectively requires emotional discipline.

Healthcare professionals often work under significant pressure—high patient loads, long hours, and multiple responsibilities. In such conditions, maintaining calm is not always easy.

However, the ability to remain composed is critical.

Consider Nurse Kavita, who is approached by an angry caregiver questioning the delay in medication. The caregiver's tone is sharp and accusatory.

If Nurse Kavita reacts emotionally, the situation may escalate.

Instead, she takes a brief pause, regulates her tone, and responds calmly:

"I understand your concern. Let me check the status of the medication and update you."

This pause—often just a few seconds—creates space between reaction and response.

Staying calm does not mean suppressing emotion. It means choosing a response rather than reacting impulsively.

Setting Boundaries Without Escalation

While empathy is essential, boundaries must also be maintained.

Anger does not justify disrespectful or abusive behavior. Healthcare professionals must ensure that interactions remain respectful and safe.

The key is to set boundaries without confrontation.

Consider a situation where a patient begins using inappropriate language.

A calm response might be:

"I want to help you, but I need us to speak respectfully so we can resolve this."

This statement is firm but not aggressive. It redirects the interaction without escalating it.

A Practical Scenario: From Conflict to Resolution

Scenario One

A patient approaches the counter angrily about a delay. The staff responds defensively. Voices rise. Other patients observe. The situation becomes tense.

Scenario Two

The same situation begins with anger. The staff member listens without interruption, acknowledges the concern, and provides a clear explanation with a timeline.

The patient's tone gradually softens. The interaction becomes constructive.

The difference lies not in the issue, but in the handling of the moment.

Action in Practice: Building De-escalation Skills

Handling angry patients is a skill that can be developed through practice.

Training sessions can include role plays where participants simulate high-pressure interactions. One person plays an angry patient, while another practices responding calmly.

Feedback can focus on tone, body language, and choice of words.

Another useful practice is reflection. After a difficult interaction, professionals can ask:

- ✓ *Did I listen fully before responding?*
- ✓ *Did I acknowledge the patient's concern?*
- ✓ *Did I maintain a calm tone?*

This reflection helps build awareness and improvement over time.

The Role of Team Support

Managing difficult situations should not fall on individuals alone.

A supportive team environment allows staff to seek assistance when needed. If a situation escalates beyond control, involving a senior staff member can help restore balance.

Clear protocols for escalation ensure that staff feel supported and patients receive appropriate attention.

The Ripple Effect of Effective De-escalation

When anger is handled well, the impact extends beyond the immediate interaction.

The patient feels heard and respected. The environment remains calm. Other patients observe a system that responds with professionalism.

Conversely, poorly handled anger can create a ripple of tension across the facility.

De-escalation, therefore, is not just about resolving one situation. It is about maintaining the overall atmosphere of care.

Closing Reflection

Anger in healthcare is inevitable. It arises from fear, pain, uncertainty, and sometimes from genuine system gaps.

The challenge is not to eliminate anger, but to respond to it with skill and composure.

When handled with patience, empathy, and clarity, even the most difficult interactions can be transformed.

What begins as confrontation can become understanding. What begins as frustration can lead to resolution.

In those moments, the true professionalism of healthcare is revealed—not in clinical expertise alone, but in the ability to remain human under pressure.

And in that humanity, trust is rebuilt—one interaction at a time.

Chapter 16:
When Mistakes Happen

From Error to Integrity: Rebuilding Trust When It Matters Most

---

No healthcare system, however advanced, is completely free from error. Medicine is practiced by human beings, within complex systems, under pressure, and often with incomplete information. Mistakes may occur in diagnosis, communication, medication, documentation, or coordination.

What defines a professional system is not the absence of mistakes—but how those mistakes are handled.

When errors are hidden, denied, or minimized, they erode trust rapidly. When they are acknowledged with honesty and handled with responsibility, they can paradoxically strengthen trust.

This chapter addresses one of the most sensitive and defining aspects of professionalism: owning mistakes and communicating them with integrity.

The Natural Instinct: To Protect or To Admit

When something goes wrong, the immediate instinct for many professionals is self-protection.

There may be fear of blame, legal consequences, damage to reputation, or loss of credibility. In such moments, silence or partial disclosure may seem like the safer option.

However, from the patient's perspective, lack of transparency feels like betrayal.

Let us consider Dr. Arvind Rao, who realizes that a medication dosage prescribed earlier was higher

than intended. The patient experienced mild side effects but is now stable.
Dr. Rao faces a choice. He can avoid mentioning the error and continue treatment, hoping the issue does not surface. Or he can address it openly.
If the patient later discovers the mistake—through another doctor or through records—the sense of trust is broken, not only because of the error, but because of the lack of honesty.
In contrast, when errors are acknowledged early, with clarity and responsibility, the conversation becomes one of accountability rather than concealment.

The Cost of Hiding Mistakes

Hiding errors may seem to reduce immediate discomfort, but it often creates larger consequences.
Patients and caregivers are perceptive. Inconsistencies in communication, unexplained changes in treatment, or defensive responses can raise suspicion.
Consider Mrs. Leela Menon, whose husband experiences an unexpected reaction after a procedure. When she asks for an explanation, she receives vague answers from different staff members.
Her concern shifts from the medical issue to the lack of clarity. She begins to question the system itself. What could have been a manageable situation becomes a trust crisis.
Transparency does not eliminate the seriousness of an error. But it prevents the additional damage caused by uncertainty and doubt.

Owning the Error: A Professional Responsibility

Owning a mistake requires courage, clarity, and structure.

It is not about assigning blame or over-explaining. It is about acknowledging what happened, explaining its impact, and outlining the steps being taken to address it.

Let us revisit Dr. Rao's situation.

Instead of avoiding the conversation, he speaks to the patient:

"I want to discuss something important with you. I reviewed your previous prescription and realized that the dosage was higher than it should have been. I'm sorry for this error. The good news is that we have identified it early, and I have already adjusted the medication. I will continue to monitor you closely to ensure everything is stable."

This approach does three things. It acknowledges the error, takes responsibility, and provides reassurance about corrective action.

The patient may still feel concerned, but the presence of honesty creates a foundation for trust.

The Role of Apology in Healthcare

An apology in healthcare is not merely a formality. It is a recognition of impact.

Patients do not expect perfection, but they do expect accountability. A sincere apology acknowledges that something went wrong and that it mattered.

However, apologies must be handled carefully. A vague or defensive apology can do more harm than good.

Consider two responses.

"I'm sorry if there was any confusion."

This shifts responsibility away from the professional and minimizes the issue.

Now consider:

"I'm sorry for the mistake that occurred. I understand that this may have caused concern, and I take responsibility for addressing it."

The second response is clear, direct, and accountable.

An effective apology does not weaken authority. It strengthens credibility.

A Practical Framework for Apology

While every situation is unique, a structured approach can help professionals navigate these conversations. The process begins with a clear acknowledgment of what happened. This must be factual and free from ambiguity.

It is followed by an expression of regret—not as a formality, but as a genuine recognition of the impact.

Next comes an explanation, in simple terms, of what led to the error. This should not be overly technical or defensive.

Finally, the focus must shift to action—what is being done to correct the issue and prevent recurrence.

Let us consider Nurse Deepa, who administered a medication later than scheduled due to a coordination lapse.

When speaking to the patient, she says:

"I want to let you know that your medication was delayed earlier due to a coordination issue. I'm sorry for that. I have now ensured that your schedule is back on track, and I will personally monitor it to prevent this from happening again."

The clarity and ownership in this response restore confidence.

Managing the Emotional Response

When mistakes are disclosed, patients and caregivers may react with concern, frustration, or even anger.

This is a natural response.

The role of the healthcare professional is not to control the reaction, but to respond to it with patience and openness.

Consider Mr. Thomas, who becomes visibly upset when informed about an error in his test scheduling. Instead of becoming defensive, the staff member listens and says:

"I understand why this is upsetting. Let me explain what happened and how we are correcting it."

By acknowledging the emotion, the conversation moves from confrontation to resolution.

Creating a Culture Where Errors Can Be Addressed

Handling mistakes effectively is not just an individual responsibility. It requires a supportive system.

In environments where staff fear punishment or blame, errors are more likely to be hidden. In environments that encourage reporting and learning, errors become opportunities for improvement.

Consider a hospital that introduced regular review meetings—not to assign blame, but to understand system gaps.

Staff began to report issues more openly. Processes were refined. Over time, the frequency of certain errors reduced.

The shift was not in perfection, but in openness and learning.

A Scenario: Two Different Outcomes

Scenario One

An error occurs. It is not communicated clearly. The patient becomes aware through indirect means. Trust is broken. The situation escalates.

Scenario Two

The error is identified and communicated promptly. The professional acknowledges it, apologizes sincerely, and outlines corrective steps.

The patient feels concerned but respected. Trust is maintained.

The difference lies in transparency and ownership.

Action in Practice: Building Confidence in Difficult Conversations

Professionals often hesitate to disclose errors because they lack confidence in handling the conversation.

Training can play a critical role here.

Role plays can simulate scenarios where participants practice acknowledging mistakes and delivering apologies. Feedback can focus on clarity, tone, and emotional responsiveness.

Reflection is equally important. After any incident, professionals can ask:

- ✓ *Was I clear in acknowledging the issue?*
- ✓ *Did I take responsibility?*
- ✓ *Did I provide reassurance about next steps?*

Over time, this builds confidence and consistency.

The Strength in Accountability

There is a common misconception that admitting mistakes reduces authority.

In reality, the opposite is true.
Patients are more likely to trust professionals who are transparent and accountable. They recognize honesty as a sign of integrity.
When handled well, a difficult moment can become a defining one—where trust is not only preserved but strengthened.

Closing Reflection

Mistakes are an inevitable part of complex systems. But how they are handled defines the character of those within the system.
When errors are hidden, trust erodes quietly but deeply. When they are acknowledged with honesty and addressed with responsibility, trust is rebuilt.
In those moments, professionalism is not measured by perfection, but by integrity.
And in healthcare, where trust is the foundation of every interaction, integrity is not optional.
It is essential.

Chapter 17:
Conflict Between Staff & Patients

When Systems Fail, People Clash

Conflict in healthcare rarely begins as conflict.

It often starts as a small gap—an unanswered question, a delayed response, a miscommunication between departments, or a missing piece of information. Left unaddressed, these gaps widen. Frustration builds quietly. Assumptions take over. And eventually, what began as a system issue surfaces as a human confrontation.

By the time it becomes visible, it appears as a clash between staff and patient. Voices rise. Positions harden. Emotions take control.

This chapter explores a critical but often overlooked truth: most conflicts are not caused by difficult people, but by broken communication within the system.

Understanding this changes everything. It shifts the focus from blaming individuals to strengthening processes, from reacting to conflict to preventing it.

Where Conflict Really Begins

Let us consider Mr. Dinesh Varadarajan, admitted for a minor surgical procedure. The doctor informs him that he will be discharged the next morning.

The next day arrives. By noon, there is no update.

Mr. Dinesh approaches the nurse, who says, *"Please check with billing."* Billing says, *"We are waiting for the doctor's note."* The doctor, meanwhile, assumes the paperwork is already initiated.

By 2:00 p.m., Mr. Dinesh is frustrated.

He returns to the nursing station, this time with a sharper tone. *"Why is this taking so long? Nobody seems to know anything!"*
From the staff's perspective, they are doing their part. From the patient's perspective, the system is failing him.
The conflict that follows is not about attitude. It is about lack of coordination.

The Domino Effect of Internal Breakdown
In healthcare settings, departments are interdependent. A delay in one area affects another.
When communication between teams is unclear or inconsistent, the patient becomes the point where all gaps converge.
Consider Mrs. Farida Sheikh, waiting for a diagnostic report. The lab has completed the report but has not updated the system. The doctor is unaware that it is ready. The receptionist continues to tell the patient to wait.
Mrs. Sheikh grows increasingly anxious.
Eventually, she raises her voice at the reception desk, saying, *"I've been waiting for hours! What is happening?"*
The receptionist, unaware of the internal delay, feels unfairly targeted. Now both sides feel frustrated. This is the domino effect of internal breakdown. The patient experiences the system as one unit. Any disconnect within that unit becomes visible as conflict.

Recognizing the Early Signs of Conflict
Conflict rarely appears suddenly. It builds in stages.
A patient begins by asking questions. When answers are unclear, the tone changes. When the issue

persists, frustration becomes visible. If still unresolved, it escalates into confrontation.

Healthcare professionals who recognize these early signs can intervene before escalation.

Let us consider Ravi, who approaches the front desk multiple times asking about his test results. Each time, he receives a brief response: *"Not yet."*

By the third interaction, his tone becomes sharper.

If the staff recognizes this as an early signal and responds with more clarity—"*The report is expected by 4 p.m., and we will inform you as soon as it is ready*"—the escalation can be prevented.

Early intervention is not about solving the entire problem immediately. It is about acknowledging and guiding the situation before it intensifies.

When Conflict Surfaces: The Immediate Response

Despite best efforts, some conflicts will still surface.

When they do, the first response is critical.

Consider Mr. Joseph, who raises his voice at a nurse about a delay in medication. The nurse feels defensive and responds sharply. The situation escalates quickly.

Now imagine a different response.

The nurse pauses, maintains a calm tone, and says, *"I understand your concern. Let me check the status of your medication and update you immediately."*

This response does not deny the issue. It does not challenge the emotion. It redirects the interaction toward resolution.

In moments of conflict, the goal is not to assert authority. It is to restore calm and regain control of the situation.

The Role of Escalation Protocols

One of the most important tools in managing conflict is a clear escalation protocol.

When staff members are unsure of how to handle a situation, or when a conflict exceeds their level of authority, there must be a structured way to involve the right person.

Consider a hospital where staff are trained to escalate issues in a defined manner.

If a patient is dissatisfied at the front desk, the concern is first addressed by the receptionist. If unresolved, it is escalated to a supervisor. If still unresolved, a senior administrator or patient relations officer steps in.

This structured approach ensures that issues are handled at the appropriate level, without unnecessary delay or confusion.

Now contrast this with a setting where no such protocol exists. Staff members hesitate, pass responsibility, or attempt to manage situations beyond their capacity.

The result is inconsistency and prolonged conflict.

Escalation is not a sign of failure. It is a sign of system support.

A Practical Scenario: Two Systems, Two Outcomes

Scenario One

A patient is upset about a delay. The receptionist attempts to handle it but lacks authority. The issue is passed informally between staff members. No one takes ownership.

The patient becomes more frustrated. The situation escalates.

Scenario Two

The same issue arises. The receptionist listens and attempts to resolve it. When it requires further action, it is escalated to a supervisor who provides clarity and takes responsibility.

The patient feels heard and guided. The situation stabilizes.

The difference lies in clarity of process and ownership.

Bridging Internal Communication Gaps

To prevent conflict, internal communication must be strengthened.

Departments must not operate in isolation. Information must flow clearly and consistently.

Consider a simple practice implemented in a busy hospital ward.

At the start of each shift, a brief coordination meeting is held. Updates are shared—pending discharges, expected reports, special cases.

This ensures that everyone is aligned.

As a result, when patients or caregivers ask questions, staff provide consistent answers.

This reduces confusion and prevents conflict.

Action in Practice: Creating a Conflict-Ready System

Managing conflict effectively requires preparation.

Staff must be trained not only in communication skills, but also in understanding system flow. They must know whom to approach when an issue arises, and how to escalate it appropriately.

Regular training sessions can include scenario-based exercises where participants practice handling conflicts and escalating them correctly.

Equally important is feedback. After a conflict situation, teams can review what happened.

- ✓ *Was there a communication gap?*
- ✓ *Was escalation timely?*
- ✓ *Could the situation have been prevented?*

This reflection turns conflict into learning.

The Emotional Impact on Staff

It is important to acknowledge that conflict affects staff as well.

Repeated exposure to difficult interactions can lead to stress and fatigue. If not addressed, this can impact performance and attitude.

Support systems—such as team discussions, debriefing sessions, and managerial support—help staff process these experiences.

When staff feel supported, they are better equipped to handle future situations.

The Ripple Effect of Effective Conflict Management

When conflicts are handled well, the impact extends beyond the immediate interaction.

Patients feel respected, even if the issue is not fully resolved immediately. Staff feel more confident and supported. The overall environment remains calm.

Conversely, poorly handled conflict creates tension that spreads across the facility.

Conflict management, therefore, is not just about resolution. It is about preserving the culture of care.

Closing Reflection

Conflict between staff and patients is often the visible outcome of invisible system gaps.

When communication breaks down internally, it surfaces externally.

The solution lies not in controlling patients, but in strengthening systems.

Clear communication, early intervention, and structured escalation transform conflict from a disruptive force into a manageable part of healthcare.

In those moments, professionalism is not defined by avoiding difficulty, but by navigating it with clarity and composure.

And when systems support people, people respond with understanding.

That is where conflict begins to dissolve—and trust begins to rebuild.

Chapter 18:
Why Doctors Become "Insensitive"

Understanding the Erosion of Empathy in a High-Pressure System

---

It is easy to label a doctor as "insensitive."

A patient feels unheard. A caregiver feels dismissed. A consultation feels rushed, mechanical, distant. The conclusion seems obvious—the doctor does not care.

But the reality is more complex, and often more uncomfortable.

Most doctors do not enter the profession lacking empathy. In fact, many begin their journey with a strong desire to help, to heal, to make a difference. Over time, however, something changes. The tone becomes sharper. The patience reduces. The connection weakens.

This chapter does not excuse unprofessional behavior. It seeks to understand what erodes empathy, so that it can be rebuilt intentionally.

Because unless the system understands why sensitivity is lost, it cannot restore it.

The Gradual Shift: From Idealism to Survival

Let us consider Dr. Neeraj Menon, who began his career with energy and purpose. During his early years, he spent time explaining conditions to patients, answering questions patiently, and following up with genuine concern.

Over the years, his workload increased. Patient volume grew. Administrative demands multiplied. Emergencies became routine.

Gradually, his consultations became shorter. His responses became more direct, sometimes abrupt.
He did not decide to become less empathetic. He adapted to survive.
What changed was not his intention, but his capacity.
This shift is rarely sudden. It happens quietly, over time.

Burnout: When Energy Runs Out

Burnout is not simply tiredness. It is a state of emotional, physical, and mental exhaustion caused by prolonged stress.
In healthcare, burnout is common because the demands are constant and the stakes are high.
Consider Dr. Kavitha Iyer, who works long hours in a busy hospital. She sees dozens of patients each day, handles emergencies, and manages administrative responsibilities.
At the end of the day, she feels drained—not just physically, but emotionally.
When a patient asks multiple questions late in the day, her response is shorter than it would have been earlier.
It is not that she does not care. It is that her emotional reserves are depleted.
Burnout reduces the ability to engage, to listen, and to respond with patience.

Compassion Fatigue: When Caring Becomes Heavy

Compassion fatigue is different from burnout, though they often overlap.
It occurs when continuous exposure to suffering begins to affect the caregiver's emotional response.

Consider Dr. Ahmed, who works in a critical care unit. Every day, he deals with severe illness, uncertainty, and sometimes loss.

In the beginning, each case affected him deeply. Over time, to cope with the emotional intensity, he begins to distance himself. He becomes more clinical, more detached.

This detachment is not indifference. It is a protective mechanism.

Without it, the emotional burden could become overwhelming.

However, when this detachment extends too far, it appears as insensitivity.

System Overload: When Time Becomes the Enemy

Modern healthcare systems often operate under pressure—high patient volumes, limited time, and increasing expectations.

Consider Dr. Ramesh, who has a waiting room full of patients. Each patient deserves attention, but time is limited.

If he spends extended time with one patient, others wait longer. If he reduces consultation time, the quality of interaction suffers.

He is constantly balancing speed and care.

In such environments, communication becomes compressed. Eye contact reduces. Listening becomes selective.

The system, not just the individual, shapes behavior.

When systems prioritize volume over experience, empathy becomes difficult to sustain.

The Invisible Load: Beyond the Patient Interaction

Doctors carry more than what is visible in the consultation room.

They think about previous cases, upcoming procedures, administrative tasks, and personal responsibilities. They make decisions that carry significant consequences.

This cognitive load affects how they engage in each interaction.

Consider Dr. Priya Sharma, who has just completed a complex case. As she moves to the next patient, her mind is still processing the previous situation.

The next patient begins to speak, but her attention is divided.

The patient perceives this as disinterest.

In reality, it is mental overload.

A Scenario: Two Perspectives

Scenario

Mr. Anand, a patient, explains his symptoms. The doctor listens briefly, asks a few questions, and writes a prescription without much explanation.

Mr. Anand leaves feeling dismissed.

From his perspective, the doctor was insensitive.

Now consider the doctor's perspective.

He has already seen 25 patients that morning. He is running behind schedule. An emergency case is waiting. His focus is on diagnosing quickly and managing time.

He does not intend to dismiss the patient. He is operating under constraint.

Both perspectives are valid. The gap lies in experience versus intention.

Recognizing the Signs Within Oneself

For healthcare professionals, awareness is the first step toward change.

Signs of reduced empathy may include shorter responses, impatience with questions, avoidance of emotional conversations, or a sense of detachment.

These are not signs of failure. They are signals.

Recognizing them early allows for correction before they become habitual.

Rebuilding Sensitivity: Small but Intentional Shifts

Restoring empathy does not require dramatic changes. It begins with small, conscious actions.

A brief pause before responding. A moment of eye contact. A simple acknowledgment of the patient's concern.

Consider a doctor who, despite a busy schedule, begins each consultation with a short pause and a direct greeting.

"Tell me what's been troubling you."

This simple shift creates space for connection. Over time, such practices become natural, even within a busy environment.

Action in Practice: Protecting the Human Side

To sustain empathy, both individual and system-level actions are needed.

At an individual level, doctors must recognize the importance of rest, reflection, and boundaries. Continuous work without recovery leads to depletion.

At a system level, organizations must address workload, provide support structures, and recognize the emotional demands of the profession.

Peer discussions, mentoring, and even brief debriefing sessions after intense cases can help process emotional load.

Empathy is not an unlimited resource. It must be maintained and replenished.

A Training Reflection: Walking Both Sides

In training sessions, participants can be asked to reflect on two roles.

First, as a patient who felt unheard. What did that experience feel like?

Second, as a doctor under pressure. What constraints were present?

This dual perspective creates understanding.

It shifts the narrative from blame to balance.

The Responsibility That Remains

Understanding the causes of insensitivity does not remove responsibility.

Patients still experience the interaction as it is. Their perception is shaped by what they receive, not by the constraints behind it.

Therefore, even within limitations, the responsibility to communicate with respect remains.

The goal is not perfection. It is conscious effort.

Closing Reflection

Doctors do not become insensitive overnight. It is a gradual process shaped by burnout, emotional fatigue, and system pressure.

But just as sensitivity can erode, it can also be rebuilt.

Through awareness, intentional practice, and supportive systems, the human side of healthcare can be preserved.

Because at the heart of medicine is not only knowledge, but connection.
And when that connection is maintained, even in the most demanding environments, healthcare remains what it is meant to be—
Not just a science of treatment, but an art of care.

Chapter 19: Managing Stress & Emotional Exhaustion

Protecting the Caregiver to Sustain Care

There is a quiet assumption in healthcare that those who care for others must simply endure.

Long hours, emotional intensity, unpredictable situations, and constant responsibility are treated as part of the profession. Over time, this endurance becomes a habit. And slowly, without notice, stress accumulates—not as a single event, but as a continuous undercurrent.

Emotional exhaustion does not always appear dramatically. It shows up in subtle ways. A shorter response. A reduced capacity to listen. A sense of detachment. A feeling of being "on duty" even when off work.

This chapter is not about eliminating stress—that is unrealistic in healthcare. It is about managing it deliberately, so that professionals can sustain both performance and humanity.

Because when the caregiver is depleted, care itself begins to suffer.

Recognizing Emotional Exhaustion in Real Time

Let us consider Dr. Mehul Shah, who has been working extended shifts in a high-volume setting. He does not feel overwhelmed in a dramatic sense. He continues to function, to diagnose, to treat.

But small changes begin to appear.

He feels irritated when patients repeat questions. He prefers shorter interactions. At the end of the day, he feels mentally drained, yet unable to switch off.

This is emotional exhaustion—not collapse, but gradual depletion.

The challenge is that many professionals do not recognize this state until it affects their behavior.

Awareness is the first step. Noticing the shift allows for intervention before it becomes burnout.

The Nature of Stress in Healthcare

Stress in healthcare is not only about workload. It is about responsibility, unpredictability, and emotional exposure.

A doctor may move from a routine consultation to a critical case within minutes. A nurse may manage multiple patients with different needs simultaneously. A technician may work under time pressure with little margin for error.

This constant switching demands both cognitive and emotional energy.

Consider Nurse Latha, who manages a busy ward. Throughout her shift, she responds to patient needs, coordinates with doctors, handles documentation, and addresses caregiver concerns.

By mid-shift, her body is still active, but her mind feels stretched.

This is not unusual. It is the reality of the profession.

The question is not whether stress exists. It is how it is managed in the moment.

Micro-Techniques: Small Interventions with Immediate Impact

In high-pressure environments, long breaks are not always possible. This is where micro-techniques become valuable.

These are brief, practical actions that can be applied within seconds or minutes, without disrupting workflow.

Consider a simple pause between consultations.

After completing one patient interaction, instead of moving immediately to the next, the doctor takes a brief moment—just a few seconds—to reset. A deep breath. A shift in posture. A conscious release of the previous interaction.

This small pause creates a mental boundary.

Let us look at Dr. Kavya, who began practicing this technique. Between patients, she takes a slow breath and mentally says, *"Next patient, fresh attention."*

Over time, she notices that she feels less carried over from one case to another.

This is not about relaxation. It is about resetting attention.

Breathing as a Stabilizing Tool

Breathing is often overlooked because it is constant. Yet, when used intentionally, it becomes a powerful stabilizer.

In moments of pressure, breathing tends to become shallow and rapid. This signals the body to remain in a heightened state.

By slowing the breath—even for a few cycles—the body begins to settle.

Consider Rahul, a junior doctor who feels tense during peak hours. He begins practicing a simple

pattern: inhale slowly, pause briefly, exhale slightly longer.
He does this for 30 seconds between tasks.
The external situation does not change. But his internal state becomes more controlled.
This is a micro-technique that requires no additional time—only awareness.

Emotional Boundaries: Caring Without Carrying

One of the most challenging aspects of healthcare is emotional involvement.
Professionals are expected to care deeply, yet if they absorb every emotion fully, exhaustion becomes inevitable.
This is where boundaries become essential.
Boundaries are not about detachment. They are about sustainable engagement.
Consider Dr. Anita, who works in oncology. She cares deeply for her patients, but she notices that she carries their stories home with her.
Over time, this affects her emotional well-being.
With guidance, she begins to practice a mental boundary at the end of her shift.
Before leaving, she takes a moment to acknowledge her work for the day and consciously "close" it.
"I have done what I could today. I will continue tomorrow."
This does not reduce her care. It prevents emotional overflow.
Boundaries allow professionals to care without being consumed.

The Role of Physical Reset

The body often carries stress even when the mind is focused.

Simple physical resets—stretching, adjusting posture, walking briefly—can release accumulated tension.

Consider Nurse Joseph, who spends long hours on his feet. He begins incorporating short stretches during brief pauses in his shift.

These moments are small, but they reduce physical strain and improve overall energy.

Physical and emotional states are interconnected. Addressing one supports the other.

A Practical Scenario: Two Approaches to the Same Day

Scenario One

A doctor moves continuously from one patient to another, without pause. Stress accumulates. By the end of the day, interactions become shorter and less patient.

Scenario Two

The same doctor incorporates brief resets—pausing between consultations, taking a few controlled breaths, and maintaining awareness of emotional state.

The workload is unchanged. The experience is different.

The difference lies in intentional management of energy.

Creating Personal Boundaries Within the System

Boundaries are not only emotional. They are also practical.

In many healthcare settings, professionals feel compelled to be constantly available—responding to calls, messages, and requests beyond working hours.

While flexibility is part of the profession, lack of boundaries leads to continuous stress.
Consider Dr. Rohan, who responds to patient messages late into the night. Over time, he feels unable to disconnect.
With guidance, he establishes a simple boundary.
He informs patients of specific times when he is available for non-urgent communication. Urgent concerns are directed through the hospital system.
This clarity reduces constant interruption and allows him to rest.
Boundaries are not about limiting care. They are about structuring it sustainably.

Action in Practice: Building Daily Resilience

Managing stress requires consistent, small practices rather than occasional large interventions.
A brief pause between tasks. A conscious breath during pressure. A mental reset at the end of a shift. Clear boundaries for availability.
These actions may seem minor, but their cumulative effect is significant.
Training programs can incorporate these techniques, allowing professionals to practice them in real-time scenarios.
Over time, they become part of routine behavior.

The Role of Organizational Support

While individual practices are important, the system must also support well-being.
Reasonable scheduling, adequate staffing, and recognition of effort contribute to reduced stress.
Opportunities for peer interaction—where professionals can share experiences—also play a role in emotional balance.

When the system acknowledges the human side of its workforce, individuals are better equipped to sustain their roles.

Closing Reflection

Stress in healthcare is inevitable. Emotional exposure is part of the profession.

But exhaustion does not have to be.

By recognizing early signs, applying practical micro-techniques, and establishing clear boundaries, professionals can protect their energy and maintain their capacity to care.

Because the quality of care is directly linked to the state of the caregiver.

When caregivers are supported—both by themselves and by the system—they do more than function.

They connect. They engage. They heal.

And in doing so, they preserve not only the effectiveness of healthcare, but its humanity.

Chapter 20: Rebuilding Purpose in Healthcare

Returning to the Reason You Began

There comes a point in many healthcare careers when the question quietly changes.

It is no longer, *"How do I treat this patient?"*

It becomes, often unspoken, *"Why am I doing this at all?"*

This question does not arise at the beginning. In the early years, purpose feels clear. There is energy, ambition, and a strong sense of calling. The desire to heal, to serve, to make a difference is vivid and alive.

But over time, the pressures of the system—long hours, administrative demands, difficult interactions, and emotional fatigue—begin to cloud that clarity.

Purpose does not disappear suddenly. It fades.

This chapter is about reclaiming it.

The Quiet Drift Away from Purpose

Let us consider Dr. Sanjay Iyer, who entered medicine with a deep sense of commitment. He remembers the day he received his admission letter, the pride in his family's eyes, and the belief that he would make a meaningful difference.

Years later, his days are filled with back-to-back consultations, paperwork, and constant pressure to manage time.

One evening, after a long day, he pauses and realizes something unsettling.

He is doing his work—but he no longer feels connected to it.

Nothing dramatic has happened. There has been no single event. It is a gradual drift.
This is not uncommon.
Purpose is not lost because people stop caring. It is lost because the space to remember why they care disappears.

The Original Calling: More Than a Career Choice

For most healthcare professionals, the decision to enter the field is not purely transactional.
It is influenced by a desire to help, to heal, to be useful in moments that matter.
Consider Dr. Aditi Verma, who chose medicine after witnessing a family member receive compassionate care during a difficult time. That experience stayed with her.
It shaped her idea of what a doctor could be—not just a clinician, but a presence of reassurance.
Years later, in the midst of a busy practice, that memory feels distant.
Reconnecting with purpose often begins by revisiting such moments—not as nostalgia, but as anchors of identity.

When Work Becomes Mechanical

One of the strongest indicators of lost purpose is when work becomes purely mechanical.
Consultations are completed efficiently. Decisions are made accurately. But something is missing—the sense of meaning.
Consider Dr. Rakesh, who sees patients continuously throughout the day. His diagnoses are correct, his prescriptions appropriate.
Yet, he feels a sense of monotony.

Patients begin to feel like cases. Interactions become transactional.

This is not a failure of competence. It is a disconnection from purpose.

Reconnecting Through Reflection

Rebuilding purpose begins with reflection.

Not in a theoretical sense, but in a practical, personal way.

A simple question can initiate this process:

"Why did I choose this profession?"

For some, the answer may come quickly. For others, it may take time.

Consider Dr. Neha, who begins journaling at the end of her day. She writes about one patient interaction that stood out—not necessarily the most complex, but the most meaningful.

Over time, patterns emerge. She begins to notice that what gives her satisfaction is not just solving medical problems, but helping patients feel understood.

This awareness begins to reshape how she approaches her work.

Reflection brings clarity. Clarity restores direction.

Finding Meaning in Small Moments

Purpose is often imagined as something large—a life-saving intervention, a major breakthrough.

In reality, it is frequently found in small, everyday moments.

A patient who feels reassured after a conversation. A caregiver who expresses gratitude for clear guidance. A child who smiles after a procedure is explained gently.

Consider Nurse Meera, who once felt her work was routine. One day, a patient's family thanks her for taking the time to explain a procedure in simple terms.

That moment stays with her. She begins to realize that her role is not only to assist clinically, but to translate care into understanding.

Purpose is not always in the outcome. It is in the impact of presence.

A Practical Scenario: Two Ways of Experiencing the Same Work

Scenario One

A doctor completes consultations efficiently, focusing only on diagnosis and treatment. The day feels long and repetitive.

Scenario Two

The same doctor begins to consciously connect with each patient, even briefly—through eye contact, a question, or a moment of listening.

The workload is unchanged. The experience is different.

The second approach restores a sense of meaning.

Aligning Daily Actions with Core Purpose

Rebuilding purpose is not about making drastic changes. It is about aligning daily actions with core values.

If the purpose is to help patients feel cared for, then even within a busy schedule, small actions can reflect that.

A brief explanation. A moment of acknowledgment. A clear answer to a question.

These actions may seem minor, but they reconnect the professional with the reason they chose the field.

Creating Personal Rituals of Reconnection

Purpose is sustained through regular reminders.

Some professionals find it helpful to create simple rituals.

A moment of pause before starting the day, recalling the intention behind their work. A brief reflection at the end of the day, identifying one meaningful interaction.

Consider Dr. Arjun, who begins each day with a simple thought:

"Today, I will help at least one patient feel less anxious."

This intention shapes his interactions.

By the end of the day, he often finds that he has done more than that.

Purpose does not require grand statements. It requires consistent reminders.

The Role of Mentorship and Shared Stories

Reconnection is not always an individual journey. It can be supported by shared experiences.

Senior professionals who share their journeys—the challenges, the moments of doubt, and the ways they rediscovered purpose—create perspective.

Peer discussions, where experiences are shared openly, also help.

When professionals realize that others have faced similar phases, the sense of isolation reduces.

Purpose becomes a shared understanding, not a solitary burden.

Action in Practice: Rebuilding Purpose Intentionally

Rebuilding purpose requires deliberate effort.

Taking time to reflect on the original motivation. Identifying moments of meaning in daily work. Aligning small actions with core values. Creating simple rituals of reconnection.

Training programs can include guided reflection sessions where participants explore their motivations and experiences.

Over time, these practices help restore a sense of direction.

The Responsibility of the System

While individual effort is essential, the system also plays a role.

Environments that recognize effort, encourage meaningful interaction, and reduce unnecessary administrative burden support purpose.

When professionals feel valued, their connection to their work strengthens.

Purpose is not sustained in isolation. It is influenced by the culture of the organization.

Closing Reflection

Purpose in healthcare is not lost because the work changes. It is lost because the connection to the work weakens.

Rebuilding it does not require starting over. It requires remembering.

Remembering why the journey began. Recognizing the impact of everyday actions. Reconnecting with the human side of care.

Because at its core, healthcare is not only about treating conditions.

It is about serving people in moments that matter most.

And when that purpose is alive, even the most demanding days carry meaning.
Not because they are easy, but because they are worth doing.

Chapter 21:
Hospital Training Framework

From Insight to Practice: Embedding Professionalism into Daily Care

---

Many hospitals recognize the need for better communication, stronger patient experience, and more humane interactions. Workshops are conducted. Posters are displayed. Policies are written.

Yet, after a few weeks, old habits quietly return.

The gap is not in intention. It is in implementation.

Professionalism, empathy, and patient-centric behavior cannot be sustained through one-time training alone. They must be designed into the system, practiced repeatedly, and reinforced consistently.

This chapter provides a practical, field-tested framework to help hospitals move from awareness to lasting behavioral change—through a structured two-day workshop and a disciplined monthly reinforcement model.

Why Training Often Fails

Before designing what works, it is important to understand what does not.

In many institutions, training is treated as an event. Staff attend sessions, listen, participate briefly, and return to their roles.

There is initial enthusiasm. But without follow-up, the learning fades.

Consider CityCare Hospital, which conducted a full-day training on patient communication. Feedback was positive. Staff appreciated the session.

However, within a month, patient complaints about communication returned.

The reason was simple. The training created awareness, but the system did not support practice and reinforcement.

Behavioral change requires repetition, reflection, and accountability.

The Two-Day Workshop Model: Building the Foundation

The purpose of the two-day workshop is not to deliver information. It is to shift mindset and initiate behavior change.

It must be practical, immersive, and directly connected to real hospital scenarios.

Day One: Awareness and Realization

The first day focuses on helping participants see their work from the patient's perspective.

The session begins not with theory, but with experience.

Participants are asked to reflect on their own experiences as patients or caregivers. Many recall moments where they felt anxious, confused, or ignored.

This immediately creates connection.

The facilitator then introduces real-life scenarios—similar to those explored in earlier chapters. Waiting without information, receiving blunt communication, dealing with unclear processes.

Participants discuss these scenarios openly. They begin to recognize patterns in their own environment.

Let us consider Lakshmi, a receptionist who participates in such a session. She initially believes that delays are unavoidable and that patients must adjust.

As she listens to others describe their experiences, she begins to see how lack of communication amplifies frustration.

This realization is critical. Without it, change remains superficial.

The day continues with role-play exercises.

Participants act out common situations—handling an anxious patient, explaining delays, responding to complaints. These are not scripted performances, but realistic interactions.

Feedback is immediate and constructive.

By the end of Day One, participants do not just understand concepts. They feel the impact of their behavior.

Day Two: Skill Building and Application

The second day shifts from awareness to action.

Participants are introduced to practical tools—how to greet patients, how to listen actively, how to communicate delays, how to handle difficult situations.

Each concept is followed by practice.

Consider Ravi, a nurse who struggles with handling impatient caregivers. During the session, he practices responding to a simulated scenario.

Initially, his responses are defensive. With guidance, he learns to acknowledge concerns and provide clear information.

By the end of the session, his approach changes—not because he was told to change, but because he practiced a better way.

The day concludes with each participant creating a personal action commitment.
Not a broad statement, but a specific behavior they will implement immediately.
For example, a doctor may commit to making eye contact and allowing patients to complete their first sentence without interruption. A receptionist may commit to informing patients of expected waiting times.
These commitments create ownership.

Bridging the Gap: From Workshop to Workplace
The workshop is only the beginning.
Without structured follow-up, even the best training loses momentum.
This is where the monthly reinforcement plan becomes essential.
The Monthly Reinforcement Plan: Sustaining Change
Behavioral change requires consistency. The monthly reinforcement plan ensures that learning is revisited, practiced, and embedded.
Week One: Reflection and Review
In the first week after training, teams gather for a short session.
Participants share their experiences.
What worked? What was challenging? Where did they struggle?
Consider Anita, who committed to explaining procedures more clearly. She shares that while she tried, time pressure made it difficult.
This opens a discussion. Others share similar challenges. Solutions are explored collectively.
Reflection turns individual effort into shared learning.
Week Two: Focused Skill Practice

In the second week, a specific skill is selected for reinforcement.

For example, communication of delays.

Staff practice this skill in short role plays during team meetings.

The goal is not perfection, but repetition.

Over time, these behaviors become natural.

Week Three: Observation and Feedback

In the third week, supervisors or senior staff observe real interactions.

This is not an audit. It is supportive observation.

Feedback is given immediately, focusing on strengths and areas for improvement.

Consider Mr. Suresh, a front desk supervisor, who observes interactions and gently guides staff on tone and clarity.

This real-time feedback accelerates learning.

Week Four: Recognition and Reinforcement

In the fourth week, positive behaviors are recognized.

A nurse who handled a difficult situation well. A receptionist who communicated delays effectively. A doctor who demonstrated exceptional empathy.

Recognition reinforces behavior.

It signals that professionalism and patient experience are valued.

A Practical Scenario: Training That Sustains vs Training That Fades

Scenario One

A hospital conducts a one-time training. Staff return to work. There is no follow-up. Old habits return.

Scenario Two

A hospital conducts a two-day workshop followed by structured monthly reinforcement. Skills are practiced, observed, and recognized.
Over time, patient experience improves consistently.
The difference lies not in the training content, but in the continuity of effort.

Leadership's Role in Implementation
No training framework can succeed without leadership involvement.
When leaders participate in training, reinforce behaviors, and model professionalism, the impact multiplies.
Consider a hospital where senior doctors actively demonstrate respectful communication and encourage feedback.
Staff observe and adapt.
Culture is not created by policies alone. It is shaped by visible behavior at the top.

Action in Practice: Making Training a Living Process
For training to be effective, it must move beyond the classroom.
It must be integrated into daily routines, supported by leadership, and reinforced through practice.
Short, regular sessions. Real-life application. Continuous feedback.
These elements transform training from an event into a living process.

Closing Reflection
Improving professionalism and patient experience is not a one-time initiative. It is an ongoing journey.

The two-day workshop creates awareness and builds initial skills. The monthly reinforcement plan sustains and deepens them.

Together, they form a system where behavior change is not temporary, but lasting.

Because in healthcare, excellence is not achieved through occasional effort.

It is built through consistent practice, supported by structure and intention.

And when that structure is in place, professionalism becomes not an expectation—but a habit.

Chapter 22: Leadership Responsibility in Healthcare Culture

What Leaders Tolerate, Systems Become

In every hospital, there are policies, protocols, and procedures. There are manuals that describe how patients should be treated, how communication should happen, and how professionalism must be maintained.

Yet, in reality, what shapes behavior is not what is written.

It is what is seen, experienced, and tolerated.

Culture in healthcare is not created by instruction. It is created by leadership—quietly, consistently, and often unintentionally.

This chapter addresses one of the most critical truths in healthcare transformation: if leadership does not model it, the system will not sustain it.

Culture Is Not Announced. It Is Absorbed

Let us consider MetroCare Hospital, where a new policy was introduced emphasizing respectful communication and patient experience.

Posters were displayed. Training sessions were conducted. Staff were instructed to follow guidelines.

However, within weeks, old patterns returned.

Why? Because during rounds, senior doctors continued to speak abruptly. Administrators focused only on numbers—patient volume, billing, discharge rates. Feedback from patients was discussed occasionally, but not consistently.

Staff observed this.
They understood the real message: results matter more than behavior.
Culture is not what leaders say. It is what leaders consistently demonstrate.

The Silent Influence of Senior Doctors

Senior doctors hold immense influence in any healthcare setting.
Their behavior sets the tone not only for junior doctors, but for nurses, technicians, and support staff.
Consider Dr. Krishnan, a highly respected senior consultant. He is clinically brilliant, but often dismissive in communication. He interrupts patients, avoids explanations, and speaks sharply under pressure. Junior doctors observe him closely.
Over time, they begin to adopt similar patterns—not out of intention, but out of imitation.
Now consider another senior doctor, Dr. Meera Thomas, who manages her consultations with clarity and calmness. Even when under pressure, she maintains eye contact, explains briefly, and acknowledges patient concerns.
Her juniors begin to mirror this behavior.
In both cases, no formal training was given. The difference lies in what was modeled.

Administrators: The Hidden Architects of Culture

While doctors shape clinical interactions, administrators shape the environment in which those interactions occur. Their decisions influence workload, staffing, communication systems, and accountability structures.

Consider Mr. Rajiv Menon, a hospital administrator focused entirely on efficiency metrics. His daily reviews revolve around patient numbers, turnaround times, and revenue.

Patient experience is discussed occasionally, but not prioritized. Staff quickly understand that speed is valued more than connection.

Now consider Ms. Ananya Iyer, who balances operational efficiency with patient experience. In her meetings, she asks not only *"How many patients were seen?"* but also *"What was the patient feedback this week?"*

She recognizes staff who demonstrate empathy. She addresses complaints with seriousness.

The message is clear: how we treat patients matters as much as what we deliver.

Culture Setting vs Rule Enforcement

Many institutions attempt to improve behavior through rules.

- ✓ *"Be polite."*
- ✓ *"Communicate clearly."*
- ✓ *"Respect patients."*

These instructions are important, but insufficient. Rules create compliance. Culture creates consistency.

Consider a hospital where staff are instructed to greet patients. Initially, they comply. Greetings are given, but often mechanically.

Now consider a hospital where leaders themselves greet patients, engage respectfully, and expect the same from others—not through instruction, but through example.

In the second case, behavior becomes natural.

Culture is not enforced. It is internalized.

A Scenario: Two Leadership Styles, Two Outcomes

Scenario One

A hospital introduces strict guidelines for patient interaction. Staff are monitored, and deviations are pointed out.

Compliance increases temporarily. Over time, staff begin to feel pressured. Behavior becomes forced.

Scenario Two

A hospital focuses on leadership modeling. Senior doctors and administrators demonstrate respectful communication. Feedback is discussed openly. Positive behavior is recognized. Staff begin to adopt these behaviors naturally.

The difference lies in ownership versus obligation.

The Power of Consistent Messaging

Leadership must communicate priorities consistently. If patient experience is emphasized one day and ignored the next, the message becomes unclear.

Consider Dr. Arjun, who leads a department. In every team meeting, he includes a brief discussion on patient experience—one positive story, one area for improvement.

Over time, this becomes part of the department's rhythm.

Staff begin to pay attention, not because they are told to, but because it is consistently valued.

Addressing Deviations: The Leadership Test

Leadership is most visible not in routine situations, but in moments of deviation.

When a senior doctor behaves unprofessionally, how does leadership respond?

If the behavior is ignored, it becomes accepted.
If it is addressed respectfully but firmly, it sets a standard.
Consider a situation where a patient complains about a doctor's tone.
In one hospital, the complaint is dismissed due to the doctor's seniority.
In another, the issue is discussed privately with the doctor, emphasizing the importance of communication.
The second approach reinforces accountability without undermining respect.

Creating Psychological Safety for Staff

For culture to improve, staff must feel safe to speak up.
If nurses or junior doctors hesitate to point out issues, gaps remain unaddressed.
Consider Nurse Priya, who notices that patients are often not informed about delays. She wants to suggest a solution but fears being dismissed.
In a supportive environment, she is encouraged to share her observation. Her suggestion leads to a simple communication protocol.
In a restrictive environment, she remains silent.
Leadership determines whether ideas surface or stay hidden.

Action in Practice: Leadership Behaviors That Shape Culture

Leadership responsibility is not abstract. It is visible in daily actions.
A senior doctor who pauses to listen. An administrator who responds to feedback promptly. A

department head who recognizes good behavior publicly.

These actions may seem small, but they signal what matters.

Regular walk-throughs in patient areas, direct interaction with patients, and visible engagement with staff reinforce expectations.

When leaders are present and engaged, culture strengthens.

Building Accountability Without Fear

Accountability is essential, but it must be balanced.

If staff feel constantly monitored, they may comply outwardly but disengage internally.

If there is no accountability, standards decline.

The balance lies in creating a system where expectations are clear, feedback is regular, and improvement is supported.

Consider a hospital that combines observation with coaching. Staff are guided, not judged. Over time, performance improves without resistance.

The Long-Term Impact of Leadership Culture

Culture does not change overnight. It evolves through consistent leadership behavior.

When leaders model professionalism, reinforce it, and address deviations, the system aligns.

Patients begin to experience consistency. Staff feel guided and supported. The environment becomes more stable. Conversely, when leadership is inconsistent, culture becomes fragmented.

Closing Reflection

Leadership in healthcare is not limited to clinical expertise or administrative control.

It is the responsibility of shaping how care is delivered—not just technically, but humanly.

- ✓ *What leaders demonstrate becomes the standard.*
- ✓ *What leaders ignore becomes acceptable.*
- ✓ *What leaders reinforce becomes culture.*

In the end, patients may not know the policies of a hospital. But they will experience its culture in every interaction. And that culture is a direct reflection of leadership.

When leadership chooses to model respect, clarity, and empathy, the entire system begins to reflect it.

Not because it is required. But because it becomes the way things are done.

Chapter 23:
From Treatment to Healing

When Care Goes Beyond Cure

In modern healthcare, excellence is often measured by accuracy—correct diagnosis, appropriate treatment, successful procedures. These are essential. Without them, nothing else stands.

And yet, something deeper defines how patients remember their experience.

Two patients may receive identical treatment from equally competent doctors. One leaves feeling reassured, understood, and confident. The other leaves anxious, uncertain, and emotionally unsettled.

The difference is not clinical.

It is human.

This chapter explores the critical distinction between treatment and healing—and how healthcare professionals can bridge that gap consistently, even within the pressures of real-world practice.

Understanding the Difference

Treatment addresses the body. Healing addresses the person.

Treatment focuses on symptoms, diagnosis, and intervention. Healing includes emotion, understanding, reassurance, and dignity.

Consider Mr. Raghavan, who visits a hospital with chest discomfort. He is examined, tests are conducted, and he is informed that it is not a cardiac issue. He is prescribed medication and discharged.

Technically, the case is handled well. But Mr. Raghavan leaves with lingering fear. He was not told

why the pain occurred, whether it could return, or what he should watch for.
Now consider the same case handled differently.
After the diagnosis, the doctor takes a brief moment to explain the condition in simple terms, reassures him about the seriousness, and tells him what signs to monitor.
The treatment remains the same.
But in the second case, the patient experiences healing.

Why Emotional Healing Is Often Missed
Healthcare systems are designed for efficiency.
High patient volumes, time constraints, and administrative demands push professionals toward speed and precision. In such environments, emotional aspects are often seen as optional—something to be addressed if time permits.
Consider Dr. Vivek, who manages a busy outpatient department. His schedule allows only a few minutes per patient.
He focuses on diagnosis and prescription, believing that this is his primary responsibility.
Over time, he notices that patients return with repeated questions, uncertainty, and dissatisfaction.
The issue is not lack of competence. It is the absence of emotional closure.
Healing requires not more time, but more intentional use of time.

The Emotional State of Patients
Patients do not enter hospitals as neutral individuals.
They arrive with fear, confusion, and often incomplete information.

A diagnosis, even when minor, can trigger anxiety. A delay can create frustration. A lack of explanation can lead to assumptions.

Consider Mrs. Kavitha, who undergoes a routine diagnostic test. The report is delayed, and no update is provided. By the time she receives the report, her anxiety has escalated far beyond the actual medical concern.

The delay was operational. The distress was emotional.

Healing requires recognizing that every clinical interaction has an emotional dimension.

A Practical Scenario: Same Treatment, Different Experience

Scenario One

A patient is diagnosed with a manageable condition. The doctor provides a prescription and moves to the next patient. The patient leaves with unanswered questions.

Scenario Two

The doctor provides the same prescription but adds a brief explanation: what the condition means, what to expect, and when to return.

The patient leaves with clarity and confidence.

The clinical outcome is identical. The patient experience is not.

Micro-Moments That Create Healing

Healing does not require long conversations. It is often built in small moments.

A doctor who pauses for eye contact before speaking. A nurse who explains a procedure before performing it. A receptionist who acknowledges a delay with clarity.

These actions take seconds. But they change perception completely.

Consider Nurse Lincy, who works in a surgical ward. Before administering an injection, she takes a moment to say, *"You may feel slight discomfort, but it will pass quickly."*

The patient relaxes. The procedure is the same. The experience is different.

The Role of Language in Healing

Words carry weight.

Medical terminology, while precise, can create distance. Simple language creates connection.

Consider Dr. Farhan, who initially uses technical terms while explaining conditions. Patients nod, but often do not fully understand.

He begins to simplify his explanations. Instead of saying *"hypertension,"* he says, *"Your blood pressure is higher than normal, and we need to control it to protect your heart."*

Patients respond with clarity. Healing begins with understanding.

Addressing Fear Directly

One of the most overlooked aspects of healing is addressing fear.

Patients rarely express fear directly. It appears in questions, hesitation, or repeated visits.

Consider Mr. Joseph, who asks multiple questions about his medication. The doctor initially feels impatient. On closer attention, it becomes clear that the patient is not questioning the treatment—he is seeking reassurance.

When the doctor responds with patience and clarity, the repeated questioning stops.
Fear, when acknowledged, reduces. When ignored, it persists.

Creating Emotional Closure

A consultation is not complete when the prescription is written.
It is complete when the patient feels they understand their condition and the next steps.
Consider ending interactions with a simple question:
"Is there anything you would like me to clarify?"
This creates space for the patient to express concerns.
Even in a busy setting, this moment of closure makes a significant difference.

Action in Practice: Integrating Healing into Routine Care

Healing can be integrated into daily practice without disrupting workflow.
A brief explanation after diagnosis. A moment of acknowledgment at the beginning of a consultation. A clear statement of next steps at the end.
These actions do not require additional resources. They require awareness and intention.
Training programs can include exercises where professionals practice delivering both treatment and explanation within limited time.
Over time, this becomes natural.

The System's Role in Supporting Healing

While individual behavior is critical, the system must support it.

Reasonable consultation times, clear communication processes, and supportive environments enable professionals to engage meaningfully.

Consider a hospital that encourages doctors to provide brief explanations and supports this through manageable scheduling.

The result is not only better patient experience, but also fewer repeat visits due to confusion. Healing is not an individual effort alone. It is a system-supported outcome.

A Story of Transformation

At Harmony Care Hospital, patient feedback consistently highlighted a gap.

"Treatment is good, but communication is lacking."

The leadership decided to focus on integrating emotional healing into care.

Training sessions emphasized simple practices—eye contact, clear explanations, acknowledging concerns.

Within months, feedback began to change.

Patients described feeling *"heard," "understood," and "reassured."*

Clinical outcomes remained strong.

But the experience transformed.

Closing Reflection

Healthcare begins with treatment.

But it reaches its highest form in healing.

Treatment solves medical problems. Healing addresses human experience. Both are necessary.

When healthcare professionals combine clinical excellence with emotional awareness, care becomes complete. Patients do not only remember what was done. They remember how they felt. And when they feel understood, respected, and reassured, the impact of care extends far beyond the consultation. It becomes something they carry with them.

That is the difference between treating a condition and healing a person. And that is the legacy healthcare must strive to build.

Chapter 24:
Becoming a "Remembered Doctor"

What Patients Never Forget—and Why It Matters

Every doctor is remembered.

The only question is—*for what?*

Patients may not always remember the exact medication prescribed or the technical details of a procedure. But they remember something far more powerful: how they felt in your presence.

A single interaction can leave a lasting impression—sometimes for years, sometimes for life.

This chapter is not about popularity. It is about professional legacy. It is about becoming the kind of healthcare professional patients recall with trust, gratitude, and respect—rather than hesitation, discomfort, or regret.

The Reality: Memory Is Emotional, Not Clinical

Let us consider Mr. Suresh Nair, who visited two different doctors for similar complaints over a span of a few months.

The first doctor was efficient, quick, and accurate. The consultation lasted five minutes. The diagnosis was correct. The prescription worked.

But when asked later about the experience, Mr. Nair struggled to recall the doctor's name.

The second doctor was equally competent. The consultation lasted only slightly longer. But the doctor looked at him, listened without interruption, and explained the condition clearly. Months later, Mr. Nair not only remembered the doctor's name—he recommended him to others.

The difference was not expertise. It was experience.

What Patients Never Forget

Patients remember moments that stand out emotionally.

- ✓ *They remember being dismissed.*
- ✓ *They remember being spoken to harshly.*
- ✓ *They remember confusion that was never clarified.*

But they also remember something else.

- ✓ *They remember the doctor who reassured them when they were afraid.*
- ✓ *They remember the nurse who explained a procedure gently.*
- ✓ *They remember the receptionist who treated them with respect when they were anxious.*

These moments are not accidental. They are created.

A Scenario: Two Legacies

Dr. Arvind Kapoor is known for his clinical brilliance. His diagnoses are accurate, and his treatment plans are effective.

However, he is often abrupt. He interrupts patients, avoids explanations, and becomes impatient with repeated questions.

Patients come to him because they trust his expertise. But they rarely recommend him with warmth.

Now consider Dr. Daniel Joseph.

He is equally competent, but what sets him apart is how he engages with patients. He listens fully, explains clearly, and acknowledges concerns.

Patients leave his consultation not only treated, but reassured.

Years later, families still refer to him as *"the doctor who cared."*
Both doctors treated patients. Only one built a lasting legacy.

The Three Moments That Define Memory

In most patient interactions, three moments shape how the doctor is remembered.

- ✓ *The beginning, where the patient forms a first impression.*
- ✓ *The middle, where understanding and connection are built.*
- ✓ *The end, where clarity and reassurance are established.*

Consider Mrs. Latha, who visits a clinic for a persistent headache.

- ✓ *If the doctor begins the consultation without acknowledgment, she feels like a number.*
- ✓ *If the doctor interrupts her explanation, she feels unheard.*
- ✓ *If the consultation ends without clarity, she leaves uncertain.*

Now imagine the same interaction handled differently.
A simple greeting at the beginning. A few uninterrupted seconds to explain her concern. A clear explanation and closing reassurance.
The time taken is nearly the same. The memory created is entirely different.

Small Behaviors, Lasting Impact

Becoming a "remembered doctor" does not require extraordinary actions.
It is built through small, consistent behaviors.

A doctor who remembers a returning patient's concern.

A nurse who addresses a patient by name.

A professional who acknowledges discomfort before a procedure.

Consider Dr. Mehul, who makes it a habit to ask, *"How have you been since your last visit?"*

This simple question creates continuity. Patients feel seen—not just as cases, but as individuals.

Handling Difficult Moments: Where Memory Is Strongest

Patients often remember doctors most vividly during difficult moments.

A serious diagnosis. A complication. A delay. These are moments of heightened emotion.

Consider Mr. Rahman, who receives unexpected news about his health.

If the doctor communicates bluntly, without preparation, the memory becomes one of shock and distress.

If the doctor takes a moment to prepare him, explains gently, and allows space for questions, the same information is received differently.

The situation is the same. The experience is not.

Difficult moments are not just clinical events. They are defining memories.

The Risk of Negative Memory

It is important to recognize that negative experiences are remembered more strongly than positive ones.

A single dismissive interaction can overshadow multiple neutral ones.

Consider Mrs. Priya, who had generally acceptable experiences at a hospital. During one visit, she is spoken to harshly by a staff member.
That single moment shapes her overall perception. She shares this experience with others. Reputation is built slowly, but can be affected quickly.

A Practical Scenario: Two Endings
Scenario One
A consultation ends with the doctor writing a prescription and saying, *"Take these medicines."*
The patient leaves with questions.
Scenario Two
The doctor concludes by saying, "*This medication should help reduce your symptoms. If you notice any changes or have concerns, please feel free to come back. Is there anything you would like me to clarify?"*
The patient leaves with confidence.

The difference lies in closing the interaction with care.

Action in Practice: Building a Memorable Practice
Becoming a "remembered doctor" requires intention.
It begins with awareness—recognizing that every interaction contributes to memory.
It continues with consistency—ensuring that respectful communication, listening, and clarity are part of every consultation.
Training programs can include exercises where professionals reflect on their own experiences as patients.
What did they remember? What made the difference?
This reflection translates into practice.

Creating a Personal Standard

Every healthcare professional must define their own standard. Not based on external pressure, but on personal commitment.

Consider Dr. Anita, who decides that no patient will leave her consultation without understanding their condition. This becomes her standard.

Over time, it defines her reputation.

Patients begin to trust not only her expertise, but her approach.

The Role of the System

While individual behavior is critical, the system must support it.

Excessive workload, unclear processes, and lack of support can limit the ability to engage meaningfully.

Hospitals that prioritize patient experience create environments where professionals can practice these behaviors consistently.

A Story That Stays

Years later, patients rarely recall the exact details of treatment. But they remember the doctor who sat down when they were anxious.

They remember the nurse who explained a procedure gently. They remember the moment they felt understood.

These are not grand gestures. They are human moments.

Closing Reflection

Every doctor is remembered.

Not just for what they did, but for how they made people feel.

Technical skill earns respect. Human connection earns trust.
When both come together, a doctor becomes more than a professional.
They become a presence patients return to, recommend, and remember—with gratitude. And that is the true measure of a career in healthcare.
Not only in outcomes. But in the lives touched along the way.

Chapter 25:
The Future of Healthcare – Skill + Soul

Where Technology Meets Humanity

Healthcare is changing faster than ever before.

Digital records, teleconsultations, AI-assisted diagnostics, automated systems—what once seemed distant is now part of everyday practice. Efficiency has improved. Access has expanded. Accuracy, in many cases, has increased.

And yet, a quiet question remains.

As systems become more advanced, are patients feeling more cared for—or less?

The future of healthcare will not be decided by technology alone. It will be defined by how well professionals integrate skill with soul—precision with presence, speed with sensitivity, systems with human connection.

This chapter explores how to navigate that future without losing what matters most.

The Shift: From Personal Interaction to Digital Interface

Let us consider Dr. Karan Malhotra, who now conducts a significant portion of his consultations online. His schedule is efficient. Patients log in, describe symptoms, receive prescriptions, and disconnect.

Clinically, the system works.

But something is missing.

Patients often send follow-up messages—not for medical clarification, but for reassurance. They ask questions that were not asked during the consultation.

The interaction was complete. But the experience was not.

Technology has made healthcare faster. But it has also created distance.

The challenge is not to resist technology—but to humanize it.

When Efficiency Replaces Experience

Healthcare systems often prioritize efficiency—and rightly so.

Shorter waiting times, faster reporting, streamlined processes.

But when efficiency becomes the only goal, experience begins to suffer.

Consider CityPulse Diagnostics, where reports are delivered within hours through automated systems. Patients receive results quickly—but without explanation.

Many turn to the internet, misinterpret findings, and experience unnecessary anxiety.

The system is efficient. But it is not complete.

Efficiency must be balanced with interpretation and reassurance.

The Risk of Depersonalization

As technology increases, the risk of depersonalization grows.

Patients may begin to feel like data points—numbers in a system rather than individuals with concerns.

Consider Mrs. Fernandes, who visits a hospital where registration, consultation, and billing are all

automated. The process is smooth. But at no point does she feel acknowledged as a person.
No one looks at her. No one asks how she feels. She leaves with a diagnosis—but without connection.
Technology should simplify processes, not replace human presence.

A Practical Scenario: Technology Without Soul vs With Soul

Scenario One

A patient receives a digital report via SMS. The report indicates an abnormal value. There is no explanation or follow-up.
The patient becomes anxious, searches online, and assumes the worst.

Scenario Two

The same report is delivered digitally. Along with it, a brief message explains the finding in simple terms and advises the next step.
If needed, a short follow-up call is offered.
The information is the same. The experience is transformed.

The Role of the Doctor in a Tech-Driven World

As technology takes over routine tasks, the role of the doctor evolves. Doctors are no longer just providers of information. They become interpreters, guides, and stabilizers.
Consider Dr. Ayesha Khan, who uses AI-assisted tools for diagnosis. The system provides data quickly and accurately. But she understands that her role is not replaced.
She uses the time saved to engage more meaningfully with patients—explaining, reassuring, and guiding.

Technology enhances her skill. It does not replace her presence.

Humanizing Digital Consultations

Telemedicine is here to stay. But virtual consultations must not become mechanical.

Simple adjustments can restore connection. Looking directly at the camera instead of the screen.

Allowing the patient to complete their explanation without interruption. Using the patient's name. Summarizing the discussion before ending the call.

Consider Dr. Rahul, who initially struggled with virtual consultations. Patients seemed disengaged. He began to consciously apply these small changes.

Over time, patient satisfaction improved—not because the platform changed, but because the approach did.

The Emotional Gap in Technology

Technology processes information. It does not process emotion.

A machine can detect abnormalities. It cannot sense fear. A system can deliver results. It cannot reassure.

This gap must be filled by the healthcare professional.

Consider Mr. Daniel, who receives a complex report. The system flags it as "abnormal."

He feels anxious. When he consults his doctor, the explanation is calm, clear, and reassuring.

His anxiety reduces—not because the report changed, but because someone guided him through it.

Integrating Technology Without Losing Humanity

The goal is not to choose between technology and human connection.

It is to integrate both.

Technology can handle speed, data, and efficiency.

Humans provide interpretation, empathy, and reassurance.

Consider a hospital that uses digital systems for registration and reporting, but ensures that every patient interaction includes a moment of human engagement.

A greeting. An explanation. A closing reassurance.

The system becomes efficient—and human.

Action in Practice: Designing "Human Touchpoints"

In a technology-driven environment, human interaction must be intentional.

Hospitals can identify key moments where human engagement is essential.

- ✓ *At registration, where first impressions are formed.*
- ✓ *During consultation, where understanding is built.*
- ✓ *At discharge, where clarity is critical.*

Even in digital systems, messages can be designed with warmth and clarity.

Training programs must include modules on digital communication with empathy.

A Story of Integration

At CareBridge Hospital, leadership introduced advanced digital systems.

Initial feedback was mixed. Processes improved, but patients felt disconnected.

The hospital responded by redesigning interactions. Staff were trained to engage patients personally, even within digital workflows. Reports included simple explanations. Follow-up calls were introduced for critical cases.

Within months, patient feedback shifted.

Technology remained. But now, it was supported by human connection.

The Future Professional: Skill + Soul

The healthcare professional of the future must be both technically proficient and emotionally intelligent.

- ✓ *Skill ensures accuracy.*
- ✓ *Soul ensures connection.*
- ✓ *One without the other is incomplete.*

Consider a doctor who relies entirely on systems. The care becomes efficient, but impersonal.

Consider a doctor who ignores technology. The care becomes personal, but limited.

The future lies in integration.

Closing Reflection

Healthcare is evolving. Systems will become faster. Tools will become smarter. Processes will become more efficient.

But one element must remain constant. The human connection.

Patients will continue to seek not only answers, but assurance. Not only treatment, but understanding.

When technology and humanity work together, healthcare reaches its highest potential.

It becomes precise, efficient, and deeply human.

And in that balance—between skill and soul—the future of healthcare will be shaped.

Not by machines alone. But by professionals who know how to use them—without losing what makes care truly meaningful.

Chapter 26:
Role Play Modules (Ready-to-Use)

Turning Awareness into Behavior Through Practice

Training in healthcare often fails at a predictable point—the transition from understanding to doing.

Professionals may agree with concepts like empathy, communication, and professionalism. They may even feel motivated after a workshop. But when they return to the real environment—busy OPDs, anxious caregivers, time pressure—the old patterns return.

This is where role play becomes indispensable.

Role play is not about acting. It is about rehearsing reality in a safe space, so that when the real moment arrives, the response is already familiar.

This chapter provides ten ready-to-use role play scenarios drawn from everyday hospital situations. Each scenario is designed to be practical, relatable, and immediately usable in training sessions.

The intention is not to memorize scripts, but to internalize better ways of responding.

How to Use These Role Plays

Each scenario can be conducted in small groups.

One participant plays the patient or caregiver. Another plays the healthcare professional. A third observes.

The first round is performed as it typically happens—the "natural" response. The second round is performed using improved communication and behavior.

The contrast is where learning happens.

Scenario 1: The Long Wait Without Information
Situation
Mr. Krishnan has been waiting for over an hour. No updates have been provided.
First Interaction (Typical)
Patient: *"How much longer do I have to wait?"*
Receptionist: *"Please wait. Doctor is busy."*
The patient walks away frustrated, feeling ignored.
Improved Interaction
Patient: *"How much longer do I have to wait?"*
Receptionist: *"I understand the wait has been long, sir. The doctor is currently running about 30 minutes behind due to an emergency case. We appreciate your patience, and I will keep you updated."*
The delay remains, but the frustration reduces.

Scenario 2: The Doctor Who Doesn't Look Up
Situation
A patient is explaining symptoms while the doctor continues typing without eye contact.
First Interaction (Typical)
Patient speaks. Doctor types, nods occasionally, interrupts with questions. The patient feels unheard.
Improved Interaction
The doctor pauses typing, looks at the patient, and says, *"Please tell me what has been troubling you."*
After listening, the doctor resumes documentation.
This simple shift creates connection without increasing consultation time significantly.

Scenario 3: Handling an Anxious Mother
Situation
A mother brings her child with a fever. She is visibly worried.
First Interaction (Typical)

Nurse: *"Wait outside."*
No explanation is given.
The mother's anxiety increases.
Improved Interaction
Nurse: *"We will call you shortly. The doctor is attending another patient. Your child will be seen next. If you notice any changes, please let me know."*
Clarity reduces anxiety.

Scenario 4: Delivering a Difficult Diagnosis
Situation
A serious diagnosis needs to be communicated.
First Interaction (Typical)
Doctor: *"It's cancer. You need to start treatment immediately."*
The patient is shocked and overwhelmed.
Improved Interaction
Doctor: *"I would like to discuss your reports with you. The results show a serious condition. Let me explain what this means and the options we have for treatment. We will go step by step."*
The information is the same, but the delivery allows space for understanding.

Scenario 5: The Angry Caregiver
Situation
A caregiver is upset about a delay in treatment.
First Interaction (Typical)
Caregiver: *"Why is nothing happening?"*
Staff: *"We are doing our job. Please don't shout."*
The situation escalates.
Improved Interaction
Caregiver: *"Why is nothing happening?"*

Staff: *"I understand this is frustrating. Let me check the status immediately and update you."*
Acknowledgment reduces intensity.

Scenario 6: Explaining a Procedure
Situation
A patient is about to undergo a procedure and appears nervous.
First Interaction (Typical)
Staff: "*Lie down. Don't move.*"
The patient feels anxious and uninformed.
Improved Interaction
Staff: *"I will explain what we are about to do. You may feel slight discomfort, but it will be brief. If you feel uneasy, let me know."*
Information builds trust.

Scenario 7: Billing Dispute
Situation
A patient questions an unexpected charge.
First Interaction (Typical)
Patient: *"Why is this charge here?"*
Staff: *"That's the bill. You have to pay."*
The patient feels dismissed.
Improved Interaction
Patient: *"Why is this charge here?"*
Staff: *"Let me explain this for you. This charge is for the additional test that was conducted. If you would like, I can show you the details."*
Transparency reduces conflict.

Scenario 8: Internal Miscommunication Affecting Patient

Situation

A patient is sent between departments due to lack of coordination.

First Interaction (Typical)

Staff 1: *"Go to billing."*

Billing: "*Go back to the doctor.*"

The patient becomes frustrated.

Improved Interaction

Staff: *"I will coordinate this for you. Please give me a moment while I check with the doctor and billing."*

Ownership replaces confusion.

Scenario 9: Late Report Delivery

Situation

A patient is waiting for a diagnostic report.

First Interaction (Typical)

Patient: "*Is my report ready?"*

Staff: *"Not yet."*

Repeated multiple times.

Improved Interaction

Staff: *"Your report is expected by 4 p.m. We will inform you as soon as it is ready. If there is any delay, I will update you."*

Expectation is set clearly.

Scenario 10: End-of-Day Fatigue

Situation

A doctor is tired at the end of a long day. A patient asks multiple questions.

First Interaction (Typical)

Doctor: *"Just take the medicines. You'll be fine."*

The patient leaves unsure.

Improved Interaction

Doctor (even if brief): *"I understand you have questions. Let me answer the most important ones now, and if needed, we can review again."*
Even limited time can be used with intention.

Making Role Play Effective

The value of these scenarios lies not in reading them, but in practicing them.
When participants act out both the ineffective and effective versions, the difference becomes clear—not just intellectually, but emotionally.
Observers play an important role. They note tone, body language, and clarity. Feedback is given immediately, focusing on what improved and what can be refined.
Over time, these role plays build confidence.
Staff begin to respond differently—not because they are instructed to, but because they have experienced better ways of handling situations.

A Training Insight: Practice Before Pressure

In real situations, there is little time to think.
Role play allows professionals to practice responses before they are needed.
When a similar situation arises in real life, the response feels familiar.
This is how training translates into behavior.

Closing Reflection

Professionalism and patient experience are not shaped by policies alone. They are shaped by every interaction.
Role play bridges the gap between knowing and doing. It transforms abstract ideas into practical behavior.

When healthcare professionals rehearse real situations, they prepare not just for routine interactions, but for moments that matter.

And in those moments, the difference between a standard response and a thoughtful one can change the entire experience of care.

That is the power of practice.

And that is where training becomes transformation.

Chapter 27:
Assessment & Feedback Tools

Measuring What Matters, Improving What Counts

In many healthcare institutions, there is a sincere desire to improve patient experience. Training programs are conducted, policies are revised, and expectations are clearly communicated.

Yet, one critical element is often missing—measurement.

What is not measured is rarely improved consistently.

Professionalism, communication, and patient experience are sometimes treated as intangible qualities. However, they can be observed, assessed, and strengthened—when the right tools are in place.

This chapter focuses on building practical, usable systems for capturing feedback and evaluating behavior, not as a form of control, but as a pathway to continuous improvement.

Why Feedback Systems Often Fail

Before designing effective tools, it is important to understand why many existing feedback systems do not deliver results.

In some hospitals, patient feedback forms are too long, too complex, or too generic. Patients either do not fill them or provide superficial responses.

In other cases, feedback is collected but not acted upon. Staff do not see the outcome of the feedback, and over time, the process loses credibility.

Consider Green Valley Hospital, where feedback forms were placed at the exit. Most patients ignored them. Those who filled them often ticked boxes without much thought.

The management reviewed the forms occasionally, but no visible changes followed.

Gradually, the entire process became a formality.

Feedback must not become a ritual. It must become a living system that informs action.

Designing Patient Feedback That Patients Will Actually Give

Effective patient feedback begins with simplicity and relevance.

Patients are more likely to respond when the questions are clear, brief, and directly related to their experience.

Consider Mrs. Shalini Rao, who has just completed a consultation. She is willing to give feedback, but only if it is quick and meaningful.

A well-designed feedback form might ask her to reflect on specific aspects of her experience—how she was greeted, whether communication was clear, whether her concerns were addressed.

Instead of overwhelming her with too many questions, the form focuses on what matters most.

For example, after her visit, she is asked:

- ✓ *Did you feel listened to during your consultation?*
- ✓ *Were you informed about delays, if any?*
- ✓ *Was the staff courteous and respectful?*

She responds quickly because the questions are direct and relevant.

This approach increases both participation and accuracy.

Capturing the Emotional Experience

Numbers alone do not tell the full story.

A rating of "3 out of 5" does not explain why a patient felt dissatisfied.

This is where open-ended feedback becomes valuable.

After the structured questions, patients can be invited to share one positive experience and one area for improvement.

Consider Mr. Joseph, who writes:

"The doctor was very knowledgeable, but I felt rushed and could not ask all my questions."

This single sentence provides more insight than multiple ratings.

It highlights both strength and gap.

Feedback systems must create space for patient voice, not just patient scoring.

Making Feedback Immediate and Accessible

Timing plays a crucial role in feedback.

The closer the feedback is to the experience, the more accurate it is.

Hospitals can use simple methods—digital forms on tablets, QR codes, or short SMS-based surveys—to capture feedback immediately after the interaction.

Consider a clinic that introduced a quick digital feedback system at the exit.

Patients could respond in under a minute.

Participation increased significantly.

More importantly, the feedback reflected real-time experiences, allowing the team to respond quickly.

Closing the Loop: The Most Important Step

Collecting feedback is only half the process. Acting on it completes the loop.

When patients see that their feedback leads to visible improvements, trust increases.
Consider CityCare Hospital, where repeated feedback highlighted long waiting times without updates.
Instead of ignoring the pattern, the hospital introduced a simple communication protocol—regular updates in the waiting area.
Within weeks, patient satisfaction improved.
The change was not in waiting time, but in how waiting was experienced.
Closing the loop transforms feedback from data into action.

Staff Evaluation: Observing Behavior in Real Time

Just as patient feedback provides one perspective, staff evaluation provides another.
Professional behavior can be observed and assessed in everyday interactions.
However, evaluation must be structured and supportive, not punitive.
Consider Mr. Suresh, a front desk supervisor, who observes interactions between staff and patients.
Instead of making general comments, he focuses on specific behaviors.

- ✓ *Did the staff greet the patient?*
- ✓ *Was the tone respectful?*
- ✓ *Was information communicated clearly?*

These observations are noted and discussed privately.
The focus is on improvement, not criticism.

Creating Practical Evaluation Checklists

Effective evaluation checklists are simple and behavior-focused.

They do not attempt to measure everything. They focus on key actions that define patient experience.

For example, a checklist for a consultation may include:

- ✓ *Whether the doctor made eye contact at the beginning*
- ✓ *Whether the patient was allowed to complete their initial explanation*
- ✓ *Whether the diagnosis and next steps were explained clearly*

These are observable behaviors.

They can be assessed consistently.

A Scenario: Feedback Without Action vs Feedback with Impact

Scenario One

A hospital collects feedback forms regularly. Data is compiled, but no clear action follows. Staff are unaware of the results. Patients see no change.

The system loses relevance.

Scenario Two

A hospital collects focused feedback, reviews it weekly, and identifies patterns. Specific actions are taken, and staff are informed.

Patients notice improvements. Staff feel engaged.

The system becomes meaningful.

Action in Practice: Integrating Feedback into Daily Work

For feedback systems to work, they must be integrated into routine operations.

Short, regular reviews of feedback data. Quick discussions during team meetings. Immediate recognition of positive behavior. Timely correction of gaps.

Consider a department that reviews three pieces of feedback every week—one positive, one negative, and one suggestion.

This keeps the conversation active without overwhelming the team.

Over time, feedback becomes part of the culture.

Balancing Accountability and Encouragement

Evaluation must strike a balance.

If it is too strict, staff may feel pressured or defensive.

If it is too loose, it loses impact.

The goal is to create an environment where feedback is seen as support for growth, not as judgment.

Recognition plays an important role here.

When positive behaviors are acknowledged, they are repeated.

A nurse who is appreciated for clear communication is more likely to continue that behavior.

The Role of Leadership in Feedback Systems

Leadership determines whether feedback systems succeed or fail.

When leaders take feedback seriously, act on it, and communicate outcomes, the system gains credibility.

When leaders ignore feedback or treat it as a formality, the system weakens.

Consider a hospital where leadership shares monthly insights from patient feedback and highlights improvements made.

Staff see the connection between feedback and action.

This builds trust in the process.

Closing Reflection

Assessment and feedback are not about monitoring performance alone. They are about guiding improvement.

When designed thoughtfully, feedback systems provide clarity. They highlight strengths, reveal gaps, and create opportunities for growth.

In healthcare, where every interaction matters, continuous feedback ensures that professionalism and patient experience do not remain abstract ideals.

They become measurable, improvable, and sustainable.

And when that happens, care moves beyond treatment.

It becomes an experience that patients remember—for the right reasons.

Practical Toolkit: Ready-to-Use Patient Feedback Form

A feedback form must be so simple that even a tired or anxious patient can complete it in less than one minute—yet powerful enough to reveal truth.
A highly effective format is a 5-question micro-feedback model.
Instead of overwhelming patients, the hospital can use a simple scale (for example: **Excellent / Good / Needs Improvement).**
A sample real-world format:

PATIENT EXPERIENCE FEEDBACK
(1-Minute Form)
"Your feedback helps us serve you better."

- ✓ *Did you feel respected and treated courteously during your visit?*
- ✓ *Did the doctor/staff listen to your concerns fully?*
- ✓ *Were things explained to you clearly (diagnosis, next steps, delays)?*
- ✓ *Was your waiting experience managed well (communication, updates)?*
- ✓ *Overall, how would you rate your experience today?*

Followed by two powerful open-ended prompts:

- ✓ *"What did we do well today?"*
- ✓ *"What is one thing we can improve?"*

Why This Works

This structure captures:

- ✓ *Emotional experience*
- ✓ *Communication quality*
- ✓ *System efficiency*
- ✓ *Overall perception*

And most importantly, it captures voice, not just ratings.

Advanced Insight: Reading Between the Lines

Not all feedback is direct.

Consider this response from Mrs. Anita George: *"Doctor was good, but very fast."*

On the surface, this looks positive. But in reality, it signals:

- ✓ *Rushed consultation*
- ✓ *Lack of emotional connection*
- ✓ *Possible incomplete understanding*

Training must include interpreting feedback, not just collecting it.

Staff Evaluation Checklist
(Real-Time Observation Tool)

Supervisors often struggle because they "feel" something is wrong but cannot articulate it. A structured checklist solves this.

Below is a ready-to-use observational checklist:

Front Desk Interaction Checklist

Observer: ____________________________ Date: ____

During interaction, did the staff:

- ✓ *Acknowledge the patient within 10–15 seconds?*
- ✓ *Greet politely (verbal or non-verbal)?*
- ✓ *Maintain respectful tone throughout?*

- ✓ *Provide clear and complete information?*
- ✓ *Handle questions patiently (without irritation)?*
- ✓ *Communicate delays, if any?*

Final Observation:
Excellent / Good / Needs Improvement
Comments:

____

____

Doctor Consultation Checklist

Observer: ____________________

- ✓ Made eye contact at the beginning
- ✓ Allowed patient to speak without interruption
- ✓ Asked relevant questions attentively
- ✓ Explained diagnosis in simple language
- ✓ Checked patient understanding
- ✓ Maintained calm and respectful tone

Comments: ____________________

Nursing Interaction Checklist

- ✓ Introduced self (where appropriate)
- ✓ Explained procedure before performing
- ✓ Reassured patient during care
- ✓ Responded to patient concerns promptly
- ✓ Maintained dignity and privacy

Critical Insight

These checklists are not for policing.
They are for coaching.
The moment they are used as punishment tools, staff will resist.
The moment they are used for development, staff will improve.

The Weekly Feedback Review Model
(Highly Practical System)

Most hospitals collect feedback—but fail in structured review.

A simple and powerful system can be implemented:

- ✓ Every week, the team reviews only three pieces of feedback:
- ✓ One positive experience
- ✓ One negative experience
- ✓ One suggestion

Real-Life Example

At Sunrise Multispeciality Hospital, the weekly meeting included:

Positive: *"Nurse explained everything very clearly."*

Negative: *"Waited too long without updates."*

Suggestion: "*Please inform delays.*"

Action Taken: Introduced hourly waiting updates

Within two weeks: Complaints reduced significantly

This is not theory. This is execution.

Closing the Feedback Loop with Patients (Advanced Practice)

One of the most powerful, yet rarely used tools is closing the loop with the patient.

Consider Mr. Rajesh Kumar, who had complained about billing confusion.

Instead of ignoring it, the hospital calls him:

"Thank you for your feedback. We reviewed your concern and have now improved our billing explanation process."

What happens here?

The patient feels valued

Trust increases

The hospital differentiates itself

Most hospitals collect feedback.
Very few respond to it.
That is the difference between average and excellent systems.

Common Mistakes to Avoid (Critical Training Insight)

Even well-designed systems fail when these mistakes occur:

- ✓ *Feedback is collected but not shared with staff*
- ✓ *Too much data, no clear action*
- ✓ *Blaming individuals instead of improving systems*
- ✓ *Ignoring positive feedback (only focusing on complaints)*

Balance is essential. If staff only hear criticism, morale drops.
If they see recognition, behavior improves naturally.

Embedding Feedback into Culture

The ultimate goal is not forms or checklists.
It is culture. A culture where:

- ✓ *Feedback is expected*
- ✓ *Feedback is welcomed*
- ✓ *Feedback leads to action*

Consider a hospital where a nurse says:
"Please do give your feedback. It helps us improve."
That single sentence reflects a mature system.

Final Training Exercise (Powerful Workshop Activity)

Ask participants:

- ✓ *"Think of the last time you were a patient or caregiver.*
- ✓ *Did anyone ask for your feedback?*

✓ *Did it make any difference?"*

Then ask:

"What kind of feedback system would you respect as a patient?"

This reflection shifts perspective from internal process to human experience.

Closing Reflection

Measurement in healthcare is not about numbers.

It is about understanding experience.

Every feedback form filled is a voice.

Every comment written is a story.

Every observation noted is an opportunity.

When hospitals listen carefully, act consistently, and communicate transparently, feedback becomes more than a tool.

It becomes a bridge—between expectation and experience, between service and trust.

And when that bridge is strong, healthcare transforms.

Not just in outcomes. But in how people feel while receiving care.

That is the difference between treatment and true healing.

BONUS SECTION: READY-TO-USE IMPLEMENTATION TOOLKIT

From Knowledge to Daily Practice

Most training programs fail at a predictable point.
People understand what to do. They even agree with it. But when the shift begins, the OPD fills up, the phone rings, the pressure builds—and behavior slips back to habit.
This section exists to prevent that.
What you are about to read is not theory. It is a practical operating system—tools, formats, and structures that can be lifted and used immediately within a hospital, clinic, or diagnostic center.
The goal is simple: make professionalism, empathy, and patient experience visible, repeatable, and measurable.

Ready-to-Use Tool 1: Patient Communication Checklist

This is not meant to be carried physically in hand. It is meant to be practiced until it becomes instinct.
Consider Dr. Nikhil, who initially believed he communicated well. When he began using this checklist mentally, he realized he often interrupted patients within seconds.
The checklist brought awareness—and awareness changed behavior.
A complete patient interaction, when done well, has a rhythm.

- ✓ It begins with acknowledgment. A simple greeting. Eye contact. A moment that signals presence.
- ✓ It moves into listening—allowing the patient to speak without interruption, even if only for the first few sentences.
- ✓ It continues with clarification—asking focused questions without rushing.
- ✓ Then comes explanation—translating diagnosis into language the patient understands, not what the doctor prefers.
- ✓ Finally, it ends with closure—ensuring the patient knows what to do next and feels comfortable leaving.

Hospitals can print this as a small reference card or display it in consultation rooms.

Over time, it stops being a checklist.

It becomes professional identity.

Ready-to-Use Tool 2: OPD Etiquette Poster

Posters often fail because they are generic.

But when designed correctly, they become powerful reminders.

Imagine a simple poster placed in staff areas—not for patients, but for the team.

At Sunrise Clinic, a poster was introduced with just a few clear reminders:

- ✓ *"Look at the patient before you look at the screen."*
- ✓ *"Explain before you prescribe."*
- ✓ *"Never let a patient leave confused."*
- ✓ *"Delays are acceptable. Silence is not."*

Initially, staff smiled at it.

Within weeks, they began referring to it.

A nurse gently reminded a colleague, *"Please explain before sending the patient."*
The poster had moved from wall to behavior.
The key is simplicity and relevance. Not ten instructions. Just a few that matter.

Ready-to-Use Tool 3: "How to Deliver Bad News" Pocket Guide

One of the most defining moments in healthcare is the delivery of difficult news.
And yet, many professionals are never trained for it.
This pocket guide is designed to be simple enough to remember—even under pressure.
Consider Dr. Aakash, who once delivered a serious diagnosis abruptly. The patient and family were shocked, unable to process the information.
After training, he adopted a structured approach.
He began by preparing the setting—ensuring privacy, sitting down, and creating a moment of calm.
He then assessed what the patient already knew, before adding new information.
When he shared the diagnosis, he did so gradually, using simple language.
He paused.
He allowed silence.
He invited questions.
He closed by explaining the next steps, not leaving the patient in uncertainty. The information did not change. But the experience did.
Hospitals can provide this guide as a small laminated card or include it in training handbooks. Because in these moments, skill alone is not enough. Presence matters.

Ready-to-Use Tool 4: Staff Behavior Audit Sheet

Most hospitals audit systems—billing, processes, documentation.

Very few audit behavior. And yet, behavior defines experience.

Consider Mr. Thomas, a department supervisor who began using a simple observation sheet.

He did not announce audits. He observed quietly.

- ✓ *How did staff greet patients?*
- ✓ *Was tone respectful?*
- ✓ *Was information clear?*

He noted patterns—not to criticize, but to coach.

In one instance, he observed that delays were communicated inconsistently.

This led to a simple change—standardizing delay communication.

Within weeks, complaints reduced.

The audit sheet did not create fear. It created awareness and alignment.

Training Module 1: The 30-Minute Daily Huddle

Culture is not built in annual training sessions. It is built in daily conversations.

The 30-minute huddle is one of the most powerful tools for sustaining behavior.

At CareFirst Hospital, every morning begins with a short gathering.

Not long speeches. Not lectures. Just focused engagement.

The session begins with a quick reflection—one real patient experience from the previous day. It may be positive or challenging.

This is followed by a short discussion—what went well, what could improve.

Then, a single focus point is introduced for the day.

For example, *"Today, let us ensure every patient is informed about waiting time."*

The session ends with a brief alignment.

This daily rhythm creates consistency. It keeps patient experience alive in conversation, not buried in policy.

Training Module 2: Weekly Reflection Circles

While daily huddles maintain momentum, deeper reflection requires space.

Once a week, small groups can gather for open discussion.

Consider Nurse Asha, who shares her experience of handling a difficult caregiver.

Others listen, relate, and contribute.

These sessions are not about instruction. They are about shared learning.

In one such circle, a recurring issue emerged—patients feeling uninformed about procedures. This led to a simple solution: standardizing pre-procedure explanations.

The power of reflection circles lies in honesty.

When staff feel safe to speak, real issues surface. And real solutions emerge.

Certification Model: Patient Experience Excellence Certification

Recognition is a powerful driver of behavior.

When professionalism is acknowledged, it is repeated.

The certification model is designed to create aspiration and accountability.

At Harmony Healthcare, a structured certification program was introduced.

Staff were assessed not only on technical performance, but on communication, empathy, and professionalism.
Assessment included:

- ✓ *Patient feedback*
- ✓ *Observed interactions*
- ✓ *Participation in training*

Those who consistently demonstrated excellence were recognized as *"Patient Experience Champions."*
This was not a title alone. It became a standard others aspired to.
Over time, departments began competing—not for numbers, but for quality of care experience. Certification transformed behavior from obligation to pride.

A Practical Implementation Story

At Lifetime Hospital, leadership decided to implement this toolkit.
They began small.
A communication checklist. A simple poster. Daily huddles.
There was initial resistance.
"Too busy."
"Already doing this."
But leadership stayed consistent.
Within weeks, small shifts appeared.
Receptionists began informing patients about delays.
Doctors paused briefly before consultations.
Nurses explained procedures more clearly.
Patient feedback began to change. Not dramatically at first. But steadily.
Within three months, the hospital noticed something significant.

- ✓ *Fewer complaints.*

- ✓ *More appreciation.*
- ✓ *Better staff morale*.

The system had not changed. Behavior had.

Closing Reflection

Tools do not change culture. People do.

But people need tools.

Simple, practical, repeatable tools that fit into real work—not ideal conditions.

When these tools are used consistently, they create habits. Habits create behavior. Behavior creates culture. And culture defines experience.

This bonus section is not an addition to the manual.

It is the bridge between intention and reality. Because in healthcare, excellence is not achieved by knowing what to do.

It is achieved by doing it—every day, in every interaction.

About the Author
'GERARD ASSEY'

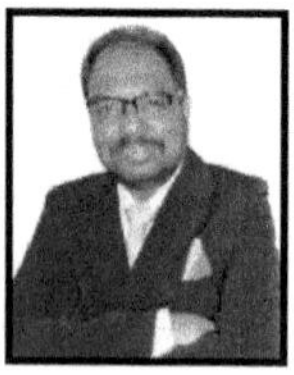

Gerard Assey is a Graduate in Economics, a PGD in Management (HRD) and holds a Doctorate in Leadership. Gerard holds several International Qualifications in Sales, Debt Collection, Training & Teaching, and is a 'Fellow' of the prestigious 'Institute of Sales & Marketing Management'-UK, a Certified NLP Practitioner, a 'Certified Trainer', an 'Accredited Management Teacher-Behavioral Sciences', a 'Certified Competency Facilitator', a 'Certified Management Consultant'- (the International credentials of a professional management consultant, awarded in accordance with global standards of the ICMCI); and a Certification from the University of Michigan in 'Successful Negotiation: Essential Strategies and Skills'

He is also a Member of the 'National Association of Sales Professionals' backed with several years experience in varied industries, both in India and Overseas. He also holds an 'Etiquette Consultant' Certification from the USA (by Sue Fox, Author of Best Seller: 'Business Etiquette for Dummies'. She has trained some of the top celebrities' world over). He was also a recipient of a scholarship for extensive training in Japan on 'Corporate Management for India'.

Gerard Assey is 'Founder & Chief Corporate Trainer' of the Group: '**Citius, Altius, Fortius Unlimited**'- an organization that **celebrated 20 years of Glorious Service** in 2021, focusing on 3 Core Competencies:

People. Performance. Profit; in functional areas of Sales & Marketing, HR & Organizational Development, covering Recruitment, Training & Consultancy!

Having managed organizations with large Sales Forces in India & Overseas, his specialization cover extensive areas of Sales Training (All levels - Presentation, Negotiation, Key/ Strategic Accounts Management & Managerial Skills for all sectors), Bid Proposal/ Capture Planning/ Management Trainings, Retail Sales, Customer Service & Customer Retention Programs, Training for Prevention & Collection of Debt, Self & Personal Development Programs (Time Management, Teamwork & Team Building, Business Etiquette & Personal Grooming, Leadership & Managerial Skills, People Management Skills, Train-the-Trainer etc), including preparation of Custom-designed Business Manuals for Internal (HR, Induction, and Sales etc) & External use (Instruction, User Manuals).

Gerard has successfully conducted over 6520 Trainings & Workshops (as of April '26) all across India, Middle East, Africa, Europe & S.E. Asia. Besides public programs conducted regularly, both in India & Overseas, he has some of the top names as clients whom he services from Single Owners to large Public & Government undertakings, covering all sectors, for their in-house needs.

His website: www.CollectionSkills.com is the only one in this part of the world to be featured in the 'Collections & Credit Risk Magazine-USA' under 'Who's Who in Training' and ranks TOP, along with other websites listed below on most search engines.

Gerard is author of 227 Books already (Apr 2026), all the books being available on all online platforms and outlets as E-books and Paperbacks

A few of our business related books:

1. Bite-sized Bits on Commonsense Management
2. Heart to Heart on Life's Principles'
3. How to become a Successful Manager
4. The Sales Professionals' Master Workbook of S.Y.S.T.E.M.S
5. The Professional Business Email Etiquette Handbook & Guide
6. The Professional Business Video-Conferencing Etiquette Handbook & Guide
7. Professional Presentation Skills
8. Exceptional Customer Service
9. Professional Tele-Marketing Skills
10. Professional Debt Collection Skills
11. The G.R.E.A.T. Sales & Service Workbook
12. Sales Training Advantage for Results (*The Ultimate Sales Training Manual to enable you stand out as a S.T.A.R.*)
13. CEO Daily Planner & Organizer
14. The Sales Professionals' Master Daily Planner
15. The Professional Debt Collector's Master Daily Planner
16. My Daily Planner & Organizer
17. MY EMERGENCY INFORMATION RECORD (Family Emergency & Peace of Mind Planner)
18. The Ultimate Therapist & Counselors Planner and Organizer
19. Building an Ethical Workplace
20. Managing Relationships at Work
21. Managing Business Meetings Effectively
22. Effective Delegation Skills
23. Goal Setting for Success
24. B2B Selling by Email
25. Professional Business Etiquette & Grooming
26. Dining Etiquette & Table Manners
27. Effective Networking Skills
28. Grooming, Etiquette & Manners for Teens, Young Adults & Future Leaders
29. Inter-Personal Skills
30. Get Ready, Get Hired!
31. Selling in a Recession
32. Effective Receivables Management in an Economic Downturn!
33. Real Estate & Property Sales Training
34. Credit Sales & Accounts Receivable Management

35. Selling Skills for Real Estate & Property Advisors
36. Take G.R.E.A.T. C.A.R.E!
37. Spa, Salon & Health Club Selling Skills
38. Selling Travel, Holiday & MICE Services
39. Selling Skills for Spa's, Salons & Health Clubs
40. Retailing in Salons & Spas
41. Selling Holiday, Vacation, Tours & Packages
42. The Power of Sales Referrals
43. Selling Luxury
44. Technical Selling Skills
45. Financial Advisors Sales Training
46. Dealing with Burnout at Work Monopolize Your Markets
47. Selling to Affluent Customers
48. Growing up with Grace
49. Financial Selling Skills
50. *The Effective Manager's Guide: Key Skills to Thrive*
51. From Aspiring to Inspiring: A Guide for New Managers on the Rise
52. The Power of Focus
53. Selling with Integrity: Sell Like Jesus The Perfect Role Model!
54. 31 Habits of Champions: Your 31-Day Journey to Greatness
55. Rejecting Grasshopper Talk: From Grasshopper to Giant-Killer-*Defeating Giants Daily!*
56. Navigate the AI-Powered Future of Bid & Proposals: Up-Skill to Stay Relevant with Alternative Career Paths & Opportunities
57. Hiring Sales Winners
58. Present with Impact
59. Success Unlocked: *Breaking Free from Habits that Hold You Back*
60. Complaints to Cheers, Feedback to Gold: Mastering Complaints Management
61. Thriving Together: *Cultivating Diversity, Equity, and Inclusion*
62. Coaching Skills for Sales Managers
63. Soaring to Success in Business & Leadership: Swifter, Higher, Stronger!
64. From Classroom to Podium: A Student's Guide to Powerful Public Speaking & Presentation Skills
65. Developing Self-Discipline
66. The CEO's 31-Day Power Plan: Unlocking Success through Essential Traits

67. Credibility Matters
68. A Winning Attitude
69. Bid & Proposal Management Using AI
70. Sales Forecasting: A Practical & Proven Guide to Strategic Sales Forecasting
71. Elevate & Energize: *50 Dynamic & Fun Activities for Peak Workplace Morale*
72. 'Sales SOS! Sales on Fire! *30 Days to Conquer Chaos & the Nightmares of Success!'*
73. Mastering Sales Managerial Skills: *Building High-Performing Teams & Driving Exceptional Results*
74. Eagle-Eyed Leadership: Unleashing the Power of 31 Lessons from Eagles
75. The Ultimate Employee Training Guide: *Training Today, Leading Tomorrow*
76. Being More Accountable at Work
77. Creating a Culture of Continuous Improvement
78. Effective Questioning & Listening Skills
79. The Power of Value Selling
80. The Growth Mindset
81. Mastering Professional Help Desk Skills
82. The Power to Lead with Empathy
83. Being Prepared: The Key to Unlocking Success
84. Youthful Spark-Youth Energizers, Activities and Games-Igniting the Fun in Youth
85. Ignite your Motivation for Success
86. Elevate Your Executive Presence: *Your Roadmap to Executive Excellence*
87. Smart Decisions: *Mastering Problem Solving with Strategic Solutions for Business Success*
88. Strategic Planning: *Developing and Implementing Strategic Plans to Achieve Long-Term Business Goals*
89. The Power of Stay Interviews
90. Developing G.R.I.T.
91. Adaptability
92. Diagnosis- *A Key Skill for Leadership*
93. The Burnout-Proof Salesperson: *The Master Guide to Preventing Stress & Burnout-* Strategies for Thriving in Sales
94. Learning from Failure: *Keys to Success*
95. Customer Success Management
96. Overcoming the Killers of Motivation
97. The C-Suite Code: *Mastering Skills for Executive Excellence'*

98. Dealing with Difficult Customers
99. Unlocking Your Potential: Mastering the Top 20 Life Skills for a Brighter Future
100. Nurturing Tomorrow's Leaders: *Essential Soft Skills Every Child Must Learn*
101. Lively & Fun Party Games for Seniors & Elders
102. Role Playing for Sales Champions: From Practice to Performance
103. Fun and Exciting Party Games for Kids
104. Case Studies for Sales
105. Role-Playing for Unbeatable Customer Service
106. Case Studies in Customer Service
107. Case Studies in Winning Negotiations
108. Case Studies in Management & Leadership
109. Case Studies in Human Resources & Talent Management
110. CEO Success Blueprint: The Essential Toolkit for CEOs and C-Level Executives
111. The Salesperson's Self-Coaching Guide: *Master Your Own Self-Coaching Plan for Success*
112. Overcoming Procrastination: *Your Ultimate Guide to Stop Delaying and Start Living Your Best Life*
113. When True Colors Are Exposed: *The Journey to Unmasking Humanity*
114. Life-Changing Habits for Teens: Teen Success Blueprint for a Bright Future
115. Workplace Stress-Free: *Proven Strategies to Thrive at Work and Beyond*
116. Objection Overruled: *The Ultimate Guide to Turning 'No' into 'Yes'*
117. Building Strong Teams: *A Comprehensive Guide to Team Building*
118. Ethical & Moral Leadership in Business: *Eliminating Unethical Practices & Building a Culture of Trust & Integrity*
119. Rising Strong: Building Positive: High Self-Esteem for a Fulfilling Life-*A Practical Guide for Students, Employees, Leaders & Entrepreneurs*
120 The Cheerful Mindset: Cultivating a Joyful Outlook Everyday
121. Leading Through Crisis: Case Studies on Crisis Management
122. Selling Beyond the Algorithms
123. MAGEN CAPD- Dialysis Record Journal

124. The Human Side of Healing: *A Master Manual on Professionalism, Patient Experience & Compassionate Care- From Treatment to Trust For Doctors, Nurses & Healthcare Teams*

Besides regularly contributing to business & trade journals, including international ones such as the 'Creative Training Techniques' and the 'Sales News' of the U.S.A, He is also a member of several prestigious bodies & trade associations, having participated in many Conferences & Workshops in India & Overseas.

Prior to his last assignment of leading & managing a large MNC as head, Gerard had a 3-year stint in the Middle East as a Consultant with a leading British Consultancy Firm.

As the past 'Official Country Representative' for the International Business Award- 'THE STEVIES'-(the business world's own Oscar) for about 4 years- he ensured a few Indian companies that qualify for the same every year!

Gerard can be contacted at:

Email: training@Sales-Training.in,training@CollectionSkills.com
Websites:

www.Sales-Training.in
www.EtiquetteWorks.in
www.CollectionSkills.com
www.RetailSalesTraining.in
www.SalesTrainingIndia.com
www.ManualPreparation.com
www.TrainingWithPuppets.com
www.FirstContactAcademy.com
www.SalesAndMarketingRecruiter.com

www.ingramcontent.com/pod-product-compliance
Ingram Content Group UK Ltd.
Pitfield, Milton Keynes, MK11 3LW, UK
UKHW021339190726
13845UKWH00027B/621

9 788169 340526